How to wean your baby

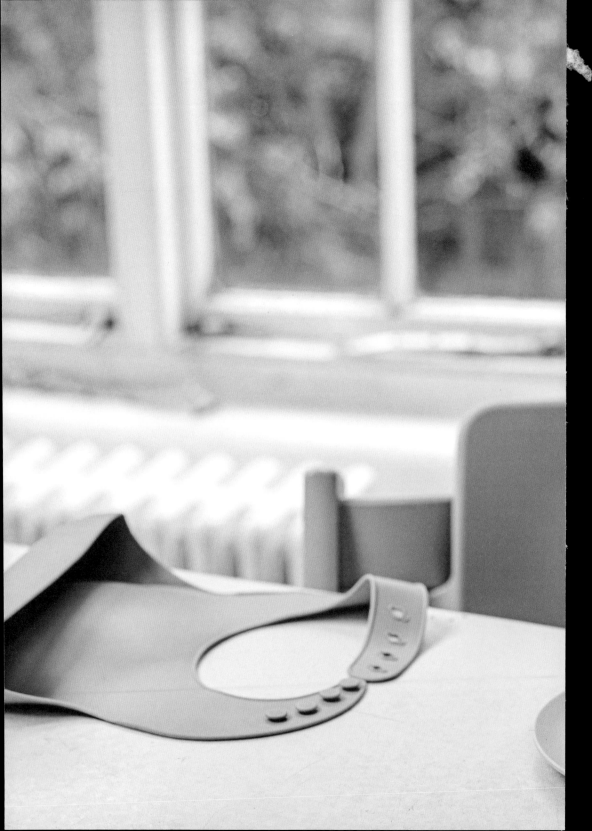

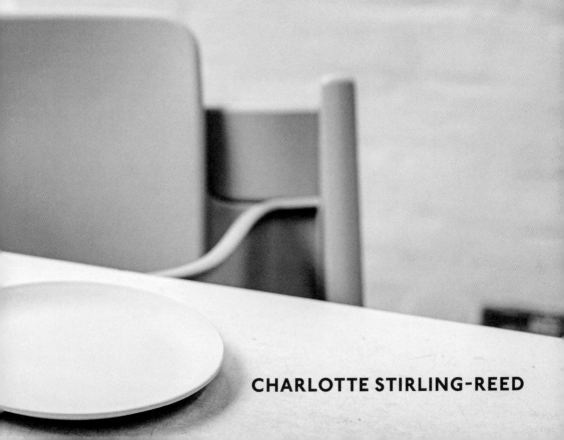

How to wean your baby

The step-by-step plan to help
your baby love their broccoli
as much as their cake

CHARLOTTE STIRLING-REED

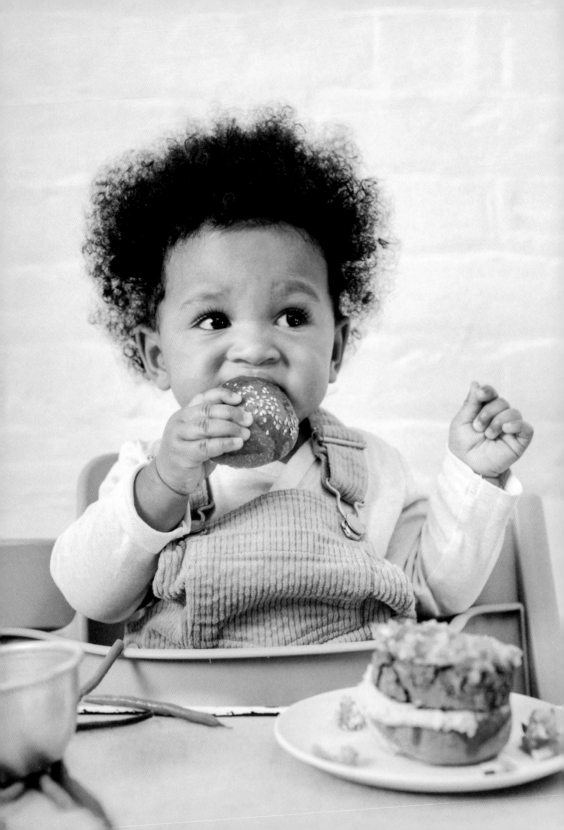

CONTENTS

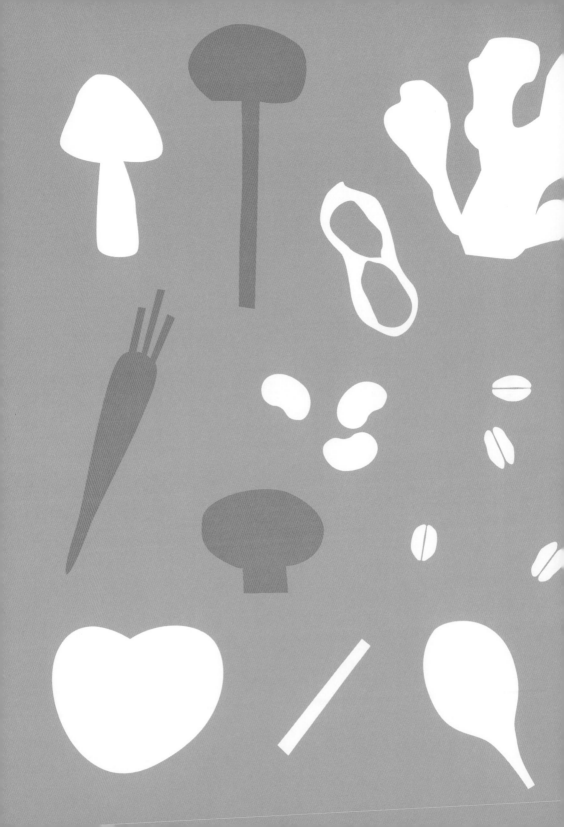

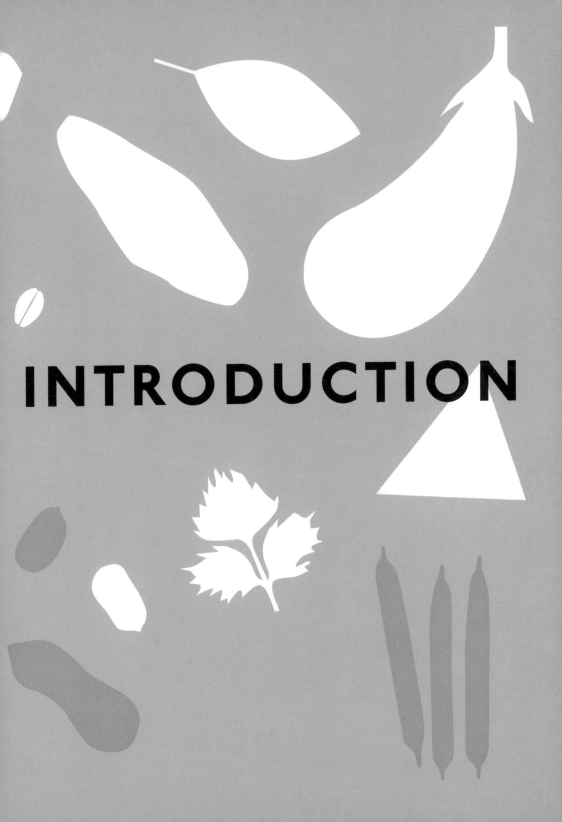

INTRODUCTION

I have spent so many years talking about the topic of weaning – it's something I speak about, think about and answer questions on every single day. You could say I live and breathe weaning!

I realised one thing from my experience of weaning my son, Raffy, as well as from talking to hundreds of parents every day: confidence is everything! So, I've made it my mission to try to boost parental confidence in feeding babies and young children.

I always feel that weaning comes at a time when, as parents, we could really do without it. At six months we're just beginning to feel we've come to terms with the lack of sleep, and feeding is often a little more structured, and finally we start to feel human again. Suddenly – BAM! – we must start considering mealtimes for babies, too.

This book aims to make this process easy and fun for new parents, so that we can enjoy raising the next generation of foodies; babies and children who are not only good little eaters, but who love food, mealtimes and eating!

I've tried to make this book as practical as possible; I'm a time-poor mum of two who is trying to juggle family life while running my own business. I don't have time to spend hours preparing gourmet recipes for my children... let's be real. That's exactly what my guide and my recipes are about – being realistic, while still raising healthy children.

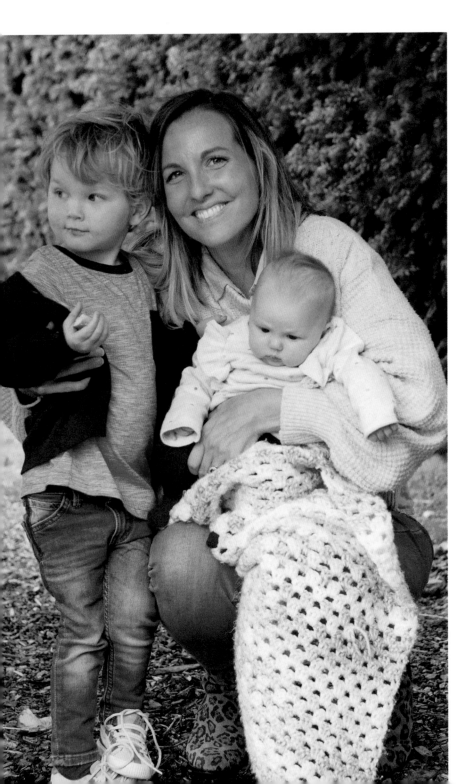

A BIT ABOUT ME

In today's connected, digital world, there are countless online experts sharing information about weaning and nutrition for children and babies; however, research or an understanding of the science of food does not always underpin their ideas.

As a registered nutritionist – with a degree in Human Biology and Nutrition and a Masters in Nutrition and Public Health – I aim to provide simple, realistic and practical advice, based on the most up-to-date research. I started my career with the UK's NHS, supporting new parents on their weaning journeys. Having since supported countless parents and having had two babies myself, I now have a real desire to share my knowledge and experience to help as many parents as possible.

Throughout this book I've used my years of first-hand practical experience, alongside my scientific understanding of child nutrition, to help you overcome the uncertainties of weaning and make your journey as enjoyable as possible. There will always be bumps along the way, but by following my advice, each step of your weaning journey will be less scary and will help set your child up for a healthy relationship with food – for life.

THE VEG-LED APPROACH

If you've followed me on social media (@SR_Nutrition) for any length of time, you'll see that I'm a big advocate of kicking off your baby's weaning journey with vegetables.

Traditionally, babies tend to be weaned on more of the sweet stuff – think fruit purees, semolina and baby rice. However, a great deal of research suggests that starting weaning by introducing vegetables first, frequently and in variety, might be a better way to go. Weaning with vegetables, and offering them in variety early on, can help to encourage an acceptance of these foods later on in life – and, let's face it, many of us need all the help we can get to encourage kids to eat up their veggies!

Weaning is about learning to taste new foods and enjoy new flavours. Babies are born with a preference for sweet foods, and breast and formula milk are both fairly sweet. However, I like to encourage people to think about weaning as a process of exploring the new, not simply reinforcing existing preferences. A baby will readily accept and gobble up the sweet stuff, certainly; but the bitter, sour and savoury tastes? They need a little help to enjoy those tastes initially, and one of the ways this works is by offering them regularly and building familiarity with those flavours early on during weaning.

MYTH BUST!

—

'I need to start my baby's weaning journey with baby rice'

This definitely isn't the case and packets of baby rice or porridge can be unnecessary and expensive. I recommend kicking weaning off with vegetables and, once you've moved through first tastes, you can offer your usual, plain porridge oats to baby.

WHY A 30-DAY GUIDE?

What I've noticed from my work over the last few years is that weaning is a challenge for many parents who are super-anxious about the little details. Yet I've also noticed that parents just need some clear guidance in the early weeks to help them become absolute pros when it comes to feeding their baby. That's why I've created a step-by-step guide to the first 30 days of weaning, starting with a veg-led approach. I know from experience that once parents have been guided through those first weeks of introducing solid foods, including what food to start with, how to introduce potential allergens etc., they will have acquired the confidence to feed their baby a beautifully varied and delicious diet, without all the stress and questions that so many parents encounter.

This guide condenses all the latest research, tips, practical hacks and my experience and knowledge, and puts them in your capable hands so can carry on your weaning journey with complete confidence.

My 5 key principles

These five key principles are important tips that I share with parents every single day. Try to keep them in mind during weaning, but also when feeding children of any age: they are crucial elements to encourage a love of food and to establish good eating habits for life.

If your little one isn't taking to solid foods as you would like – if they're starting to get a little fussy, or if you find yourself stuck in a rut with the foods you're offering – come back to these tips and make sure each of them is well and truly in place. Write them down, bookmark this page or pin the list on to your fridge.

1. Keep it calm

The more anxious you get, and the more tense mealtimes are, the more you'll find your little one doesn't really want to be a part of them. Keeping calm is often easier said than done, especially if you have a bit of an anxious personality (guilty!). However, what can really help is stepping away from the idea of getting food into your child's tummy and focusing on the idea of making the mealtime environment a nice place to be. Think about it: if you were in a situation that felt negative or unpleasant, but you couldn't escape from it, you'd soon start feeling a little reluctant to go back there day after day. If you can focus on making mealtimes an enjoyable occasion for both yourself and your little one, this can enhance the whole scenario.

Don't worry about getting your baby to eat, at first; just encourage them to be happy to sit, even if it's just to watch you eat. A bright tablecloth, some gentle music or just smiling and keeping yourself calm can make all the difference. Throughout your weaning journey, you'll notice mealtimes not going smoothly – food refusal is common (see page 120). At such times, try to pause and consider the environment that you're helping to create at mealtimes. Would you want to eat in a battleground?

2. Eat together

The simple habit of eating together is very powerful. When I speak to families who are struggling with weaning, the big mistake they often make is not eating with their little ones. Your baby will learn how and what to eat from watching you. They'll pick up cues on biting, chewing and swallowing, as well as learning how much to take and how to sip water from an open cup – all from watching you. Before you start weaning, simply bring them to the table with you and let them observe the natural behaviour of eating.

3. Always think variety

Research shows that the more variety of foods that infants are given when they are younger, the more variety they are likely to eat when they are older too. However, it's all too common to see parents doing the opposite: if baby doesn't seem to be enjoying certain foods, pulls faces or rejects something one day, they take it off the menu. Yet perhaps your baby wasn't expecting such a new taste, or didn't fancy that particular food on that occasion.

There is also plenty of evidence that babies and children need multiple offerings of certain foods before they will accept them, but also that including a variety of flavour profiles in the diet can increase a little one's liking and acceptance of foods they haven't even tasted yet (see page 34). So, don't give up offering foods to your little one just because they don't appreciate them yet. Think of all the different fruits and vegetables we have access to, as well as the adventurous foods we might not have tried ourselves yet, perhaps soya beans, millet, jackfruit...?

4. Have a routine

This one might sound boring, but it can really make a big difference to your baby's acceptance of solid foods at the start, as well as ensuring older children are hungry for their mealtimes.

Up until around six months, babies have had nothing but milk – and then, all of a sudden, they're presented with food. Babies like routine, and unless we help them to know when to expect solids and understand that there are times in the day for milk and times in the day for food, it can be a little hard for them to take to solids initially. Once they have a consistent structure where they do a similar thing (e.g. getting in the high chair) at a similar time (around lunchtime, perhaps), they quickly become more willing to accept it. It can also help you as parents to keep up with how much they've eaten and what has or hasn't gone in each day – allowing you to also think about the balance of foods they are getting at mealtimes.

5. Put eating into context

Some days baby will eat plenty, while other days they'll eat next to nothing, and that's perfectly normal. So much tends to affect your baby's appetite. It's all too easy to look at what your baby is eating from one day to the next and panic that they aren't getting enough. It's also easy to compare what your baby eats with what you see other friends' babies eating, and worry that you're getting something wrong. It's so important to remember that babies are all very different; they come with a different set of genes, with their own milestone goals and also their own appetites. If your baby's appetite takes a dive one day, take a step back and have a look at what's going on and how this might be impacting their food intake.

Avoid comparing children; some are natural grazers and eat small amounts at mealtimes, while others have huge appetites and don't ever seem to get full. The best advice is to get your little one weighed fairly regularly to ensure they are growing and developing properly. If you're ever worried, that's exactly what your health visitor and GP are there for.

How to use this book

All the information you need to set you up and prepare you for your weaning journey is in 'The basics' section on pages 16–75. If you have questions about feeding your baby and any queries on how you will deal with complications such as allergies, you'll find the answers here. The information is broken down into bite-sized chunks, with lots of infographics, charts and checklists to help keep it all simple.

Once you're feeling confident about how to begin, we enter my step-by-step guide to the first 30 days of weaning (pages 76–111). This section will offer you everything you need to breeze through your first month of weaning, including shopping lists, example meal plans and recipes.

Once you've mastered the first 30 days, the 'Next steps of weaning' (pages 112–123) shows you how to start building your own balanced meals for your baby, as well as adjusting milk amounts accordingly, and covers the all-too-common issue of food refusal.

I'll then provide you with some delicious ideas and recipes for your family meals, including breakfasts, lunches and dinners, which you can all share, as well as some finger food and lighter meal options for babies (see pages 124–197).

Finally, if you still have questions, the 'What do I do when... ?' section on pages 198–203 covers the majority of these, such as what yoghurt to give baby, what to do if baby isn't taking to weaning, and what to do if baby throws their food.

For the past few years, I've been asked by thousands of parents to produce some kind of guide to help with the weaning process – so, here it is! I really hope you enjoy How to Wean Your Baby and that it gives you the confidence to create your own little foodies. Let the weaning journey commence!

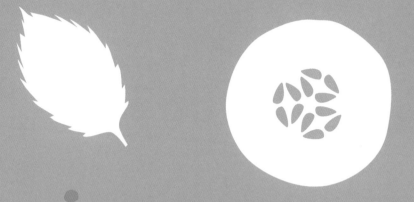

THE BASICS

1

This section is all about preparing for the weaning journey ahead so that you feel confident about each stage. You can use it like a journal, with practical tick sheets, charts and tables to help ensure the information is easy to understand and to get you involved. I'll cover everything you need to know before you start weaning. So, get stuck into these next pages for everything you need to know about successful weaning.

What is 'weaning'?

Many people still think of 'weaning' as the process of weaning baby off the breast or bottle. But weaning is all about introducing solid foods to a baby. It's sometimes called complementary feeding, reflecting the fact that this new food should be introduced alongside (not instead of!) milk.

Whenever I refer to weaning, I simply mean the process of gently introducing baby to solid foods that gradually increase in variety, amount and texture until baby is on a similar diet to the rest of the family.

WHY DO WE NEED TO WEAN?

From around six months of age, babies need more nutrition than milk alone can provide. Nutrients such as iron and zinc are starting to decline and need replacing through baby's diet. Weaning isn't just about nutrients, though: it's also about the process of learning to eat. Eating, just like walking and talking, is a skill that must be learned. Weaning is also an opportunity for baby to develop, practise and hone skills around eating. These include biting, chewing, swallowing, munching and sipping, as well as hand–eye coordination and self-feeding.

Weaning is also the process of helping babies to learn about foods, tastes and flavours. This is an opportunity to familiarise baby with a huge variety of foods. Research has shown that eating habits tend to stick: if your little one experiences a really diverse range of foods early on, they are more likely to embrace the wide variety of foods needed to make up a balanced diet later on in life.

We know that food eaten in the early years matters. The right nutrition early on in life can reduce the risk of illness and diseases throughout life, can support healthy growth and brain development, and can lead to adults who have higher IQs and go on to have healthier families themselves.

MYTH BUST!
—
'Food before one is just for fun'

Now, don't get me wrong, one of my main tips is to allow little ones to have fun with food. But food is so much more than just for fun. It's vital from six months to ensure adequate nutrition, as well as helping your child to acquire the skills to feed themselves. So, by all means have fun with food, but don't believe the myth that it's just a bit of fun – it's not.

When is my baby ready?

Until fairly recently, babies were typically introduced to solids earlier than they are now – for example, in 2005, 51 per cent of mothers had introduced solid foods by four months of age. In the UK, we recommend 'around six months of age' as a good starting point for baby's first foods. Some babies may be ready a little earlier than this, but around six months is a good estimate of when most babies will be developmentally ready. Don't worry about whether to count baby's age in months or weeks; instead, it's better to look out for their individual signs of readiness.

Use the checklist below to record signs of readiness in your baby. Look for these happening together and on multiple occasions, rather than just as one-offs:

○ **Is your baby at or coming up to six months of age?**

Date: ....

○ **Is your baby able to sit up, and hold their head and neck steady?**

Date: ....

○ **Does your baby have hand–eye coordination, so they can see an object or food and bring it to their mouth by themselves?**

Date: ....

○ **Does your baby have less of a tongue thrust reflex? (i.e. if you place your finger on their bottom lip, do they push their tongue out significantly as a reflex?) This reflex will start to lessen as your baby moves towards six months of age. A baby who is ready will swallow more than they spit out.**

Date: ....

There are plenty of other behaviours that parents often mention as signs of readiness, but many of these will just be milestone achievements for a baby at around this stage. You can always look out for some of these occurring alongside the main signs of readiness in the checklist opposite. For example, you might find that your baby:

* Takes an interest in your food and watching you eat.
* Tries to grab out for your food.
* Opens their mouth in response to you eating.
* Chews their fists and other objects.
* Wakes during the night, when previously they slept through.
* Seems hungrier than normal and unsatisfied with their usual milk.

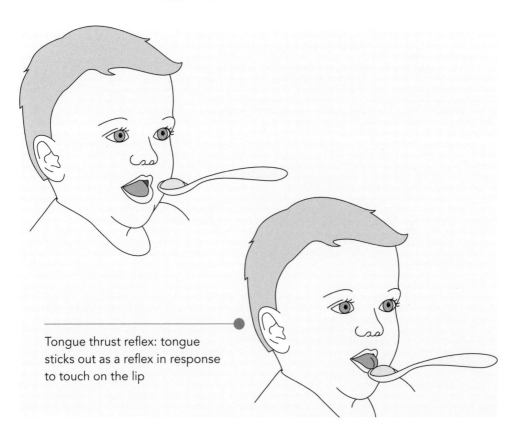

Tongue thrust reflex: tongue sticks out as a reflex in response to touch on the lip

Feeding milestones

Keeping track of developmental milestones can cause a lot of stress for parents. If your little one isn't crawling, rolling or walking when other babies of a similar age are, you can find yourself worrying that there must be something wrong. Just remember that your baby is unique and will develop at their own pace! Milestones are simply average ages when certain skills tend to become apparent – but babies will often begin, refine and ace developmental skills at totally different ages.

The timeline below summarises some of the milestones related to baby feeding. It shows the average ages, but please bear in mind that the age ranges for each milestone vary considerably.

Milestone: Suckling and swallowing
Important for?
Breast- or formula-feeding

BIRTH

Milestone:
Tongue thrust (protrusion) begins to lessen as tongue control develops
Important for?
Baby can swallow more food than they spit out – this is a sign of readiness for weaning

Milestone:
Baby begins to learn to sit unaided
Important for?
Baby can hold their trunk and focus on self-feeding and swallowing at mealtimes

AROUND 6 M

Milestone:
Gag response starts to become integrated (more like an adult's gag reflex) with exposure to food (6–12 months)
Important for?
Baby can start to control and swallow foods more effectively. Less scary for parents as the gag reflex declines

Milestone:
First teeth may begin to appear (6–12 months) although it can happen earlier
Important for?
Baby will be able to cope with slightly harder and more complex textures, with practice

Milestone:
Tongue moves forwards and backwards in the mouth
Important for?
To transfer food to the back of the mouth for swallowing

Milestone:
Mastication efficiency still developing right up until around four years
Important for?
They still might need a little modification and foods such as whole grapes and whole nuts shouldn't be offered until a child is five years

Milestone:
Can bring upper lip down to draw food off spoon.
Important for?
Baby can start to clear food from a spoon themselves

Milestone:
Baby begins to move tongue side to side in their mouth to help with munching
Important for?
Can start to use gums to flatten foods (including finger foods) before swallowing

Milestone:
Once teeth are present, can bite harder foods
Important for?
Can offer more variety of textures

Milestone:
Starts attempting use of a spoon without spilling much
Important for?
Even when spoon-feeding, you can encourage self-feeding skills

Milestone:
Pincer grip developing – baby uses finger and thumb to pick up foods (needs practice)
Important for?
You can start offering smaller pieces of foods for baby to explore and feed themselves

Milestone:
Food neophobia (fear of new foods) kicks in
Important for?
It's normal and very common for children to go through periods of food refusal

6-7 M   8+ M   9 M   12 M   14–24 M

Milk matters

Right up until one year and beyond, milk will continue to make a significant contribution to your baby's food and nutrient intakes. As you start weaning, you might notice that your baby's milk intake starts to gradually decline as their appetite for food and the amount of nutrients they get from solid food increases.

With breastfeeding, it's tricky to tell how much milk baby is getting. The advice is simply to 'feed responsively' on the basis that baby's intakes will adjust to match their needs. Once mealtimes are an established routine, you might start to notice baby spending less time on the breast and even dropping a feed or two. Carry on feeding responsively, and watch baby's signals carefully.

Responsive milk feeding means responding to signs that a baby may want to feed. These signs might include sucking fingers, wriggling, and appearing distressed, or crying. It's also about a mother's needs too, so if mum needs to feed for any reason or just wants to sit down, rest and feed baby, that's all part of feeding responsively too. Babies can be breastfed for reasons of hunger or to calm or comfort them – that's OK and breastfeeding doesn't necessarily need to fit into any particular routine.

The topic of formula milk – especially in relation to weaning – seems to be a source of great confusion. In fact, it's one of the things I'm asked about most regularly. To make it clear, I've included a graphic here that sets out the type of milk recommended at each age.

WHAT MILK, WHEN?

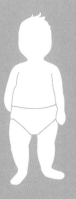

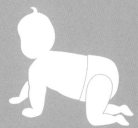

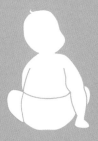

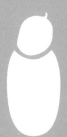

2 YRS +

At two years of age you can continue to offer breast milk as a drink to your toddler or you can offer cow's milk if you prefer. You can also switch to semi-skimmed milk once they are two as long as they have a well-balanced diet. Advice around plant milks is the same – try to choose plain and fortified options.

12-24 M

You can continue to breastfeed your baby or, if you're formula-feeding, you can switch to full-fat cow's milk as baby's main drink. Plant milks (except rice milk) can be introduced alongside a well-balanced diet (see page 26 for more on plant milks).

6-12 M

Breast or formula milk are the only milks recommended as main drinks until baby is 12 months old. However, from six months you can add full-fat cow's milk and other pasteurised plain dairy products into baby's foods and in cooking. Whole cow's milk should not be offered until one year of age as a drink. Plant-based milks (except rice drinks) can be used in cooking or mixed with food from six months. Choose unsweetened and fortified plant-based milk options.

0-6 M

Until around six months of age, babies only need breast or formula milk as a source of fluid and energy. Milk is all babies need to help them grow and develop properly. Most breastfed babies don't need any water or fluid before this, but a formula-fed baby may need a little water to drink in hot weather (see page 64).

PLANT-BASED MILKS

Just like cow's milk, plant milk alternatives should not be given as a main drink until 12 months of age. Even then, it's important to ensure they are offered as a drink alongside a well-balanced diet.

Plant-based milks such as soya, oat and almond milks (but not rice drinks, see below) can be used in cooking or mixed with food from six months, but it's important to choose options that are unsweetened. They should be fortified with calcium, and ideally, vitamin D, B vitamins and iodine too. Cow's milk contains protein, fat, energy, calcium, B vitamins and iodine and so it's important to look out for milk alternatives that at least go some way to replacing these nutrients. Plant milks vary hugely in terms of fortification (and protein and energy content), so check labels if using them.

If you want to avoid cows' milk in your little one's diet due to allergies or a desire to follow a vegan diet, it's a good idea to speak with your GP, health visitor or a registered nutritionist/dietitian first because there are important nutritional differences between plant milks and cow's milk.

Rice milks aren't recommended until a child is five years of age, due to trace levels of arsenic.

Full-fat foods for baby

It's best to offer baby full-fat dairy products, such as milk, cheese and yoghurt, and avoid low-fat products, as fat is important in a young baby's diet. Full-fat dairy can be added to foods from 6 months and baby can switch to full-fat cow's milk as a main drink from 12 months. Once baby turns two you can switch to semi-skimmed milk if your little one is eating and growing well.

HOW MUCH MILK?

Breastfeeding mums are recommended to feed responsively to mum and baby's needs (see page 24). The graph below helps to illustrate what might happen to baby's milk intakes as you move through the weaning process, and is based on formula-feeding, as it's easier to see specific amounts that a baby may be drinking. It's important to remember that the numbers shown here are just averages. Babies will all take solids and milk amounts that are individual to them, and will progress through solids at their own pace. Use the graph as a guide only so you can see how very gradually and naturally you should start to see baby's food intakes increase and milk intakes gently reduce over the first year of life.

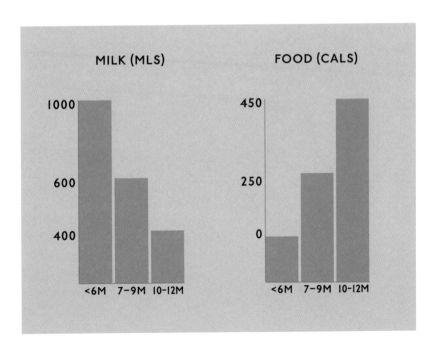

Baby-led weaning + spoon-feeding

When people begin introducing solid foods to their baby, they often feel confused about which approach they want to take: baby-led weaning or traditional spoon-feeding. The baby-led weaning (BLW) method is essentially where a baby is offered pieces of food and simply left to feed themselves from the word go – no purees or spoon involved.

THERE IS SOME RESEARCH TO SUGGEST THAT BLW MAY BE BENEFICIAL FOR:

Self-regulation of food and energy intakes

Encouraging independence around eating

Encouraging skills around self-feeding

Encouraging a positive attitude to foods and more enjoyment of eating

Less food fussiness

Earlier exposure to family-style feeding

Traditional spoon-feeding is where you offer baby some foods such as purees off of a spoon right from the start of the weaning journey.

THE BENEFITS OF TRADITIONAL SPOON-FEEDING INCLUDE:

Allows for **flexibility**

Allows a gradual introduction of solid foods including finger foods to ensure developmental readiness

Easy to modify different foods, depending on baby's needs

Potential to offer more of a variety of food which allows for a wider range of nutrients

Potential to offer a variety of textures – e.g. pureed or mashed foods off a spoon, lumpy textures, and so on

Develops skills around using utensils and spoons to feed themselves

Vary the textures

It has been shown that babies who are not exposed to textured foods until after nine months can experience more feeding difficulties. If you're following a spoon-feeding approach, it's important to start varying the texture of the foods you offer as you move through baby's weaning journey.

The combined approach

Baby-led weaning and spoon-feeding are often discussed in terms of 'either/or', which is a real shame. There is a lot of benefit to a 'best of both' approach to introducing solid foods, and the idea of a combined approach is backed by most healthcare professionals (including registered nutritionists and dietitians), supported by research findings and encouraged by the UK government.

I am a big fan of kicking off weaning by combining some purees or mashed foods with some soft cooked finger foods and just letting your little one explore. You'll soon come to realise that the first weeks – and sometimes months – of weaning are just about tiny tastes and building familiarity with the process of eating.

MYTH BUST!

—

'Offering spoons alongside BLW will confuse baby and may cause baby to choke'

There is no evidence that combining approaches confuses baby or that either approach is likely to encourage more choking. Additionally, for decades babies have been weaned with finger foods alongside purees. So don't be put off from trying a flexible, combined approach.

Some babies take to finger foods right away and love self-feeding, while others prefer a gentler journey through textures and like to use the spoon for some of their meals. Offering both methods gives your baby a chance to explore a variety of ways of feeding, so that they can figure out what and how they like to eat best. Some meals they might only want finger foods, and at other times, they might just throw them on the floor!

Just because you're spoon-feeding doesn't mean that a baby can't explore self-feeding. My son, Raffy, was adamant that he would have the spoon right away, and so we often had to load it and hand it over. He very quickly developed the coordination skills to feed himself in this way. Babies are all so different; giving them the opportunity to try a variety of methods can be helpful.

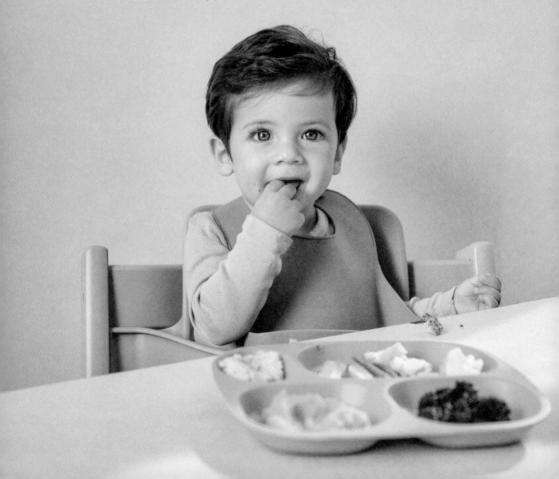

THE BENEFITS OF A COMBINED APPROACH INCLUDE:

Self-regulation

Positive eating experience

Independence

Self-feeding

Less fussiness

Variety emphasised

Baby takes the lead

Gradual approach

Family-style eating

Flexibility

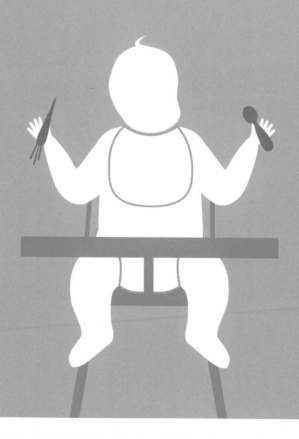

STARTING WEANING CHECKLIST

Whatever your approach to weaning, here are
some things you should check when offering your
baby their first tastes of solid foods:

Baby must be developmentally ready – not premature,
or delayed in their development in any way; if you have
any doubts, ask your health visitor.

Ensure baby is sitting up with minimal (if any) support
so they can concentrate on their arm and hand movement,
rather than trying to control their trunk.

Ensure there is an adult always present during feeding.

Finger foods offered should be soft and
manageable for a baby.

Go at baby's own pace

The initial part of weaning really is about tiny tastes. Don't
expect your baby to be gobbling up bowls of food by the
end of the first week. Babies take to weaning at different
paces, and some will only take one or two spoons or
pieces of food (if that), even after a few weeks of weaning.
This is very normal, and it's important to go at baby's
pace (see My 5 key principles on page 12).

REPEATED EXPOSURES

Research has shown that 'repeated exposures' help encourage acceptance of food. The more a baby is 'exposed' to (or offered) a food, the more familiar they are likely to become with it – and familiarity leads to acceptance.

Although I talk a lot about variety throughout this book, continuing to offer small, regular tastes of foods your baby has already tried is also important, especially if baby appears to reject them on the first few exposures.

In fact, research suggests that with some foods (especially veggies) it can take up to and beyond 10 attempts before a baby will readily accept and eat them. Therefore, once you start building in a second and third meal into baby's routine (see page 54) it's a good idea to keep repeating some of the foods that baby has already tried to help encourage more of an acceptance.

The checklist here will help you to keep track of how often your little one is having certain foods – I've listed some of those savoury and bitter vegetable options that babies often don't readily accept as good ideas to keep offering to your little one over time. Remember you don't need to offer these 10 tastes all in the first weeks or even months of weaning; just keep a note as you continue feeding your baby of how many times baby has tried them and feel free to include your own foods (maybe others that baby has rejected) to keep trying too.

Sensory feeding

When we talk about 'exposures' it doesn't have to mean baby gobbling up a whole stick of broccoli every time. Tiny tastes really do matter and even just the simple act of touching, smelling or even seeing the food is enough to 'expose' baby to a new food and encourage some kind of familiarity.

FOOD	1	2	3	4	5	6	7	8	9	10
Broccoli										
Courgette										
Avocado										
Potato										
Spinach										
Aubergine										
Cauliflower										
Swede										
Green beans										
Kale										
. . . .										
. . . .										
. . . .										

Exploring textures

If you're planning on starting with purees, you don't have to start with a super-thin puree; a thicker mash may be fine for some babies, especially if you're weaning from six months of age. However, if you prefer a more gentle approach, thinner purees are fine to start with.

Below are some visuals of textures that might work for you – pick whichever you feel comfortable with and you think your baby is ready for, and start there. It's important to move through textures fairly quickly, to allow your little one to explore and to develop the skills needed to manage more complex textures. Baby needs to have experienced a real variety of textures, including lumps, ideally by nine months of age.

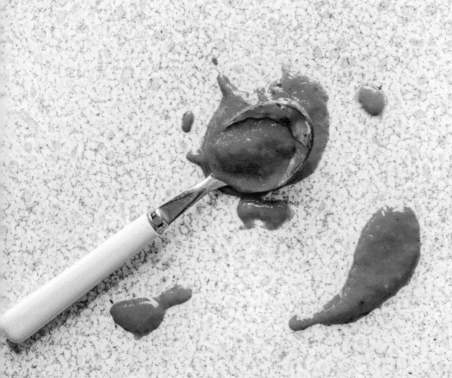

To start changing up the texture you offer
to baby, you can try three simple things when
you are prepping and cooking:

Blend less

Add less liquid

Start mashing with a fork

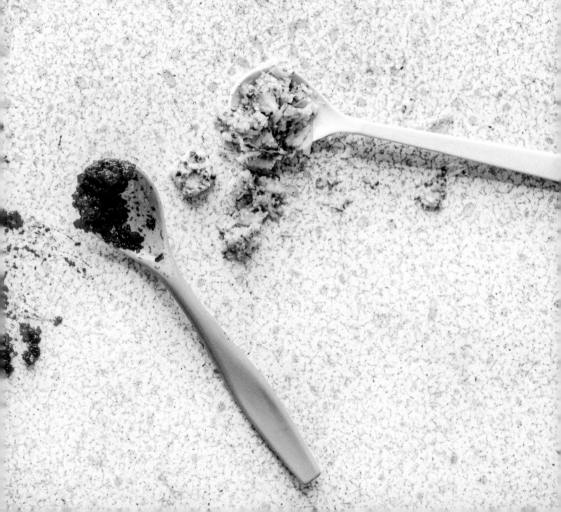

Remember that variety is key (see My 5 key principles on page 12). This holds true when we talk about textures too, so offering a variety of finger foods and textured food from a spoon can help baby to practise their skills with eating and accept more of a variety of textures later on.

Once your baby gets used to a texture and is happily swallowing it, it's good to move things up a notch. Do this gradually, so that they aren't surprised by big chunks or lumps when they've been used to thin purees. It can be a little daunting to parents to start offering chunkier and lumpier textures, but it's all about your baby learning how to cope with these – and, ultimately, exposure to new things is the best way for them to learn.

MYTH BUST!

—

'Babies without teeth can't have finger foods'

Did you know that even without teeth babies still develop the skills to chew, move food around in their mouth and swallow pieces of food? A baby's gums are pretty tough and they easily chomp and mush foods with them. So your baby doesn't need to have teeth to start enjoying textures.

This allows babies to develop and perfect the skills needed to eat like we do as an adult. Remember that babies are all different and will move at their own pace, but developmentally, these are the kind of textures your little one is likely to cope with as they move through the weaning journey.

Ideally move from pureed to chopped
gradually, over the first year of a baby's life.

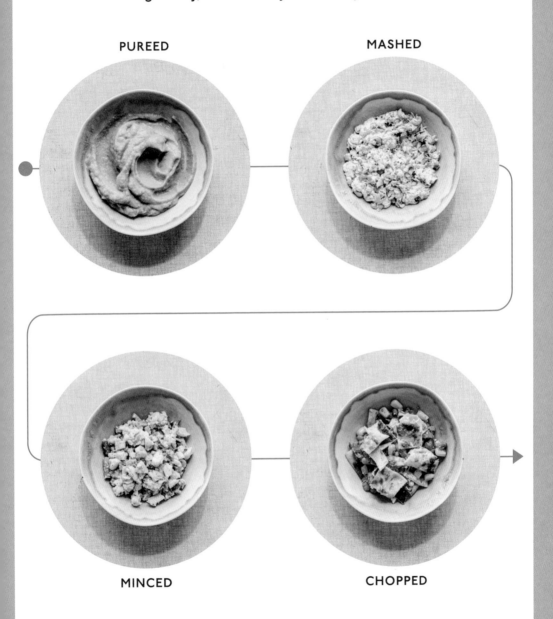

PUREED

MASHED

MINCED

CHOPPED

FINGER FOODS

Finger foods can offer more variety to your baby, get them used to new textures and let them experiment with their own skills in self-feeding (as well as lobbing foods around the kitchen, of course). Finger foods are often a cause of concern for parents – understandably! How does a baby take solid pieces of food and not choke? When it comes to finger foods, there are a few things you can do at mealtimes that can help to build both your and your baby's confidence:

✳ **Start super-soft** – think overcooked veggies, overripe fruits and super-soft cooked pasta pieces. They should easily squidge between your finger and thumb so that baby can squash these foods down with their tongue and gums.

✳ **Remove** pips, tough skins and any hard bits of the foods.

✳ **Avoid** choking hazard foods (see page 46).

✳ **Always sit with baby** when they are eating anything.

✳ **Eat** finger foods with your baby, and demonstrate yourself how to hold, how to bite off pieces and how to chew.

'They should easily squidge
between your finger and
thumb so that baby can
squash these foods down
with their tongue and gums'

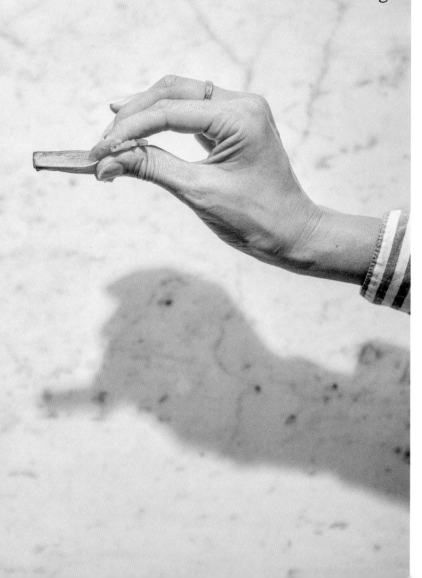

Some of my favourite finger food options include:

※ broccoli
※ cauliflower
※ sweet potato
※ kiwi fruit
※ lightly toasted bread
※ banana
※ avocado
※ pasta
※ salmon
※ courgette (skin removed)
※ large tomatoes

At the start of weaning, it's helpful to offer sticks of finger food roughly the size and shape of an adult's finger so that baby can easily grab it in their palm (they don't yet have the pincer grip) and bite off soft chunks.

Once your little one gets more confident, you can start cooking finger foods for a little less time and offering a really wide variety, so that they are gradually exposed to harder textures. Offering plenty of finger foods early on also helps to develop baby's pincer grip (see page 117).

Tip: Eating together

One thing that really helped us was showing Raffy
how to bite and chew by sitting and eating with him,
over-emphasising the chewing and biting actions myself.
Babies aren't born with an understanding of what
is an appropriately-sized piece to bite off, and so they
need to learn this from watching you!

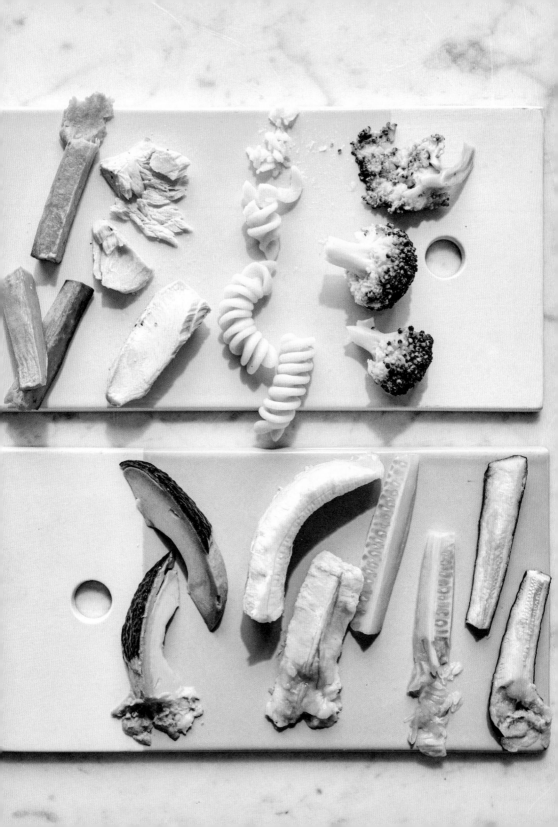

Gagging and choking

Gagging is a really normal part of your baby's weaning journey and is simply a way for a baby to remove any food that isn't ready to be swallowed. Some babies gag more than others and have quite a sensitive reflex. The gag reflex starts to lessen at around six months (see page 22) and gradually integrates so it is more similar to ours as adults. Exposure to multiple textures, including purees, lumps and finger foods, helps babies to learn how to cope with foods better and can lessen the gag response.

Choking is much less common than gagging, but it's worthwhile knowing the difference, and if you're nervous about this, I recommend doing a first aid session before your weaning journey starts.

The best things you can do to prevent choking are:

✳ **Ensure** your baby is developmentally ready for solids (see page 20).

✳ **Feed** your baby in an upright position (not at an angle or lying back in a bouncer, for example).

✳ **Always sit** with your baby when eating.

✳ **Demonstrate how** to bite, chew and swallow foods yourself.

✳ **Offer appropriate** textures and move through them gradually (see page 36).

✳ **Don't panic.**

✳ **Avoid** some of the foods that are more likely to be a choking hazard (see page 46).

✳ **Chop and prep** foods appropriately and adapt this as baby develops their skills around eating (see page 47).

GAGGING VS CHOKING

GAGGING	CHOKING

GAGGING

Tongue will thrust forward

Face may go red

You may hear spluttering,
coughing and gagging

The gag reflex is there to
keep the airway safe

Do not intervene; this can
make it worse

Let them work it out

CHOKING

Face will start to go blue

They may be quiet
or even silent

If they have an ineffective
cough or no cough at all,
shout for HELP, then start first
aid, if possible, to try to
dislodge the object

WITH THANKS TO KEEPABEAT.CO.UK FOR THIS GUIDANCE.

Choking hazards...

Here are some of the foods that
you may need to take extra precautions
with or avoid offering to your baby:

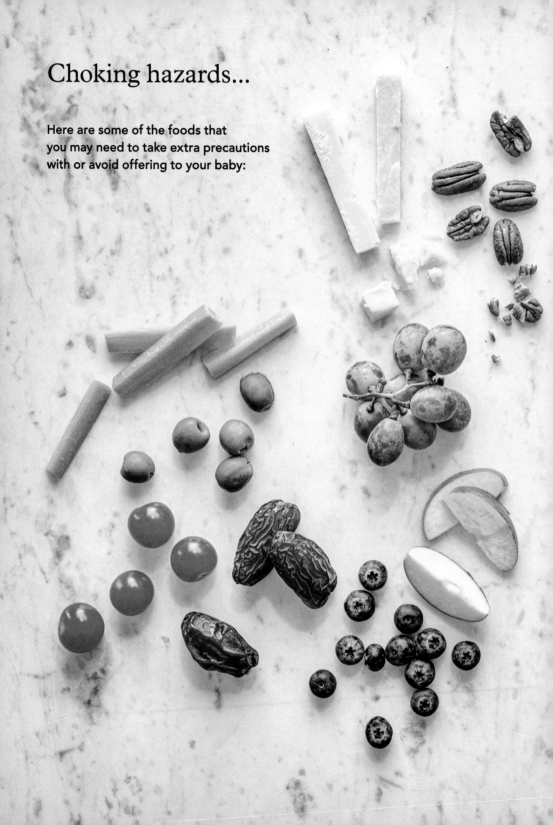

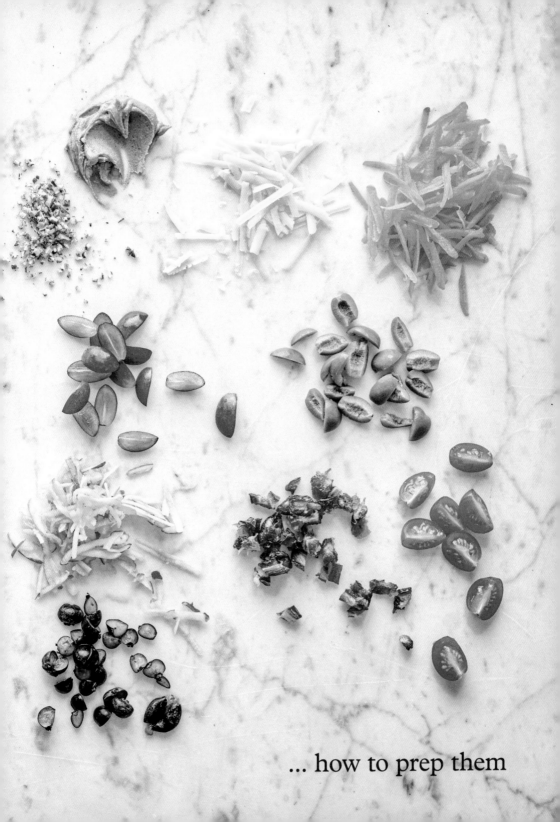

... how to prep them

Mealtime environment

It's best to choose an environment that is calm and free of distractions for baby's first meal, where they can focus on the food and enjoy the experience of you sitting down to eat together. It's also good to opt for a time of day when your little one is nice and calm. If they are too tired, hungry or distracted, their first mealtime probably won't go very smoothly.

Below are a few questions you might want to ask yourself when deciding what time of day to offer baby their first tastes of food:

When is the house at its calmest, with minimal distractions?

What's currently the calmest time of day for my baby?

When am I calmest and not rushing around?

When is there a nice gap between milk feeds and a sleep, when baby won't be too full or too tired to try something new?

Is there a time of day that a meal would fit nicely into our family routine?

The best meal to start with will vary for everyone, but once you've chosen a time of day that more or less works for you, try to stick to that time for the following days and build in a little mealtime routine around it.

Note: If your baby is at all unwell, wait until they're fully recovered before introducing solids for the first time.

Time of day to introduce allergens

When deciding on meal timings it's good to think about the fact that soon after first tastes, baby will need to be introduced to allergens – and it's recommended that these are offered earlier on in the day (morning or lunchtime at the latest), so you have plenty of time to spot a reaction and deal with it if necessary. This might mean that the first or second meal you introduce needs to be at breakfast or lunchtime. (See page 56 for more on this.)

How much should baby be eating?

Something many parents are unsure of when they start the weaning process is how much they should be giving their baby and when they should increase the portion sizes. The answer to this is complex, and there certainly aren't any specific recommendations around portion sizes for young babies. The reason for this is that babies' appetites change all the time. If they are having a growth spurt, teething, are unwell or simply tired and unhappy, it's likely their appetite will be affected. All children are individual – some are big eaters and some prefer eating smaller amounts more often.

Young children are generally good at regulating their own appetite as they tend to follow their own internal fullness and hunger signals from a young age. In fact, from birth children can regulate their own intake of milk really well, which is why responsive feeding is important during breast- and bottle-feeding, as well as weaning (see page 52).

If you're worried about how much your little one is eating – whether too much or too little – look back to my five key principles, and make sure you keep these in mind at mealtimes (see page 12).

If your baby is showing clear signs that they don't want more food (see page 53), it's always best not to attempt to force or coax them into eating more, even if it's just 'one more mouthful'. Instead, look at the bigger picture, and try to understand the reasons why your little one might not want food in that moment. They may have had enough for now; it's too close to nap time; they have just had a milk feed; they aren't feeling well; or they weren't calm at the start of the meal, for example. Respond appropriately by simply removing the food or taking baby from the high chair to do something else.

Some babies do seem to want larger portions of food, and many parents are surprised by how much their little ones eat. It's still ideal to follow their cues and allow them to have more at mealtimes if they ask for it (within reason). If your baby has a large appetite, it can help to try to slow the pace of mealtimes. You can also try:

* **Offering a smaller portion of food** initially followed by a second portion, if requested.

* **Offering a variety of textures** within a meal, which can help to slow the pace of eating.

* **Role modelling** by sitting with baby and demonstrating a slower pace of eating.

* **Teaching baby communication** signals around their appetite e.g. signalling to stop, rubbing tummy if hungry and simply asking them if they are full.

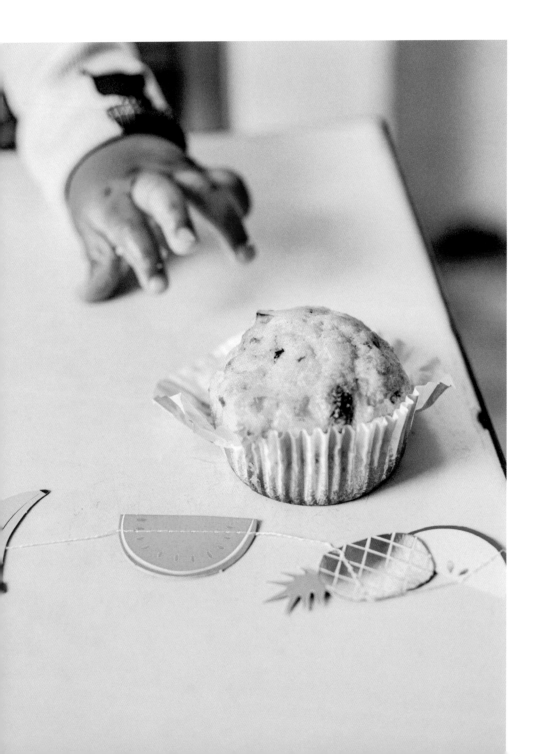

Responsive feeding

We looked at responsive feeding earlier, when thinking about milk feeds, and this continues into solid foods. With weaning, responsive feeding means:

※ **Setting up a feeding environment** which is calm and comfortable, at a time of day when baby is likely to expect and want food.

※ **Offering foods that are appropriate** for a baby at their particular developmental stage.

※ **Listening, watching and responding** to a baby's signs of hunger or fullness appropriately – offering more if it's required, or stopping the mealtime if baby has had enough.

MYTH BUST!

—

'I need a guide to portion sizes for my baby!'

No such thing actually exists as babies' appetites are all so different and change daily. Rather than having a preconceived idea of how much a baby should eat at any given meal, or when they should be hungry, it's much more about understanding that this will change frequently – from day-to-day and meal-to-meal – and adapting to baby's signals around how much they want at each meal or feed.

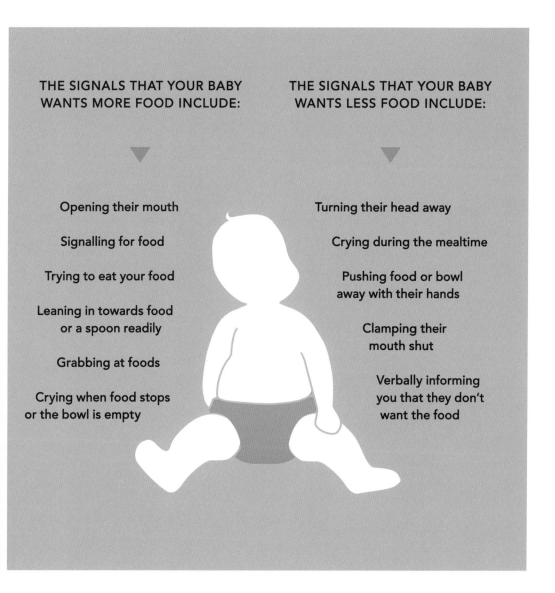

THE SIGNALS THAT YOUR BABY WANTS MORE FOOD INCLUDE:

Opening their mouth

Signalling for food

Trying to eat your food

Leaning in towards food or a spoon readily

Grabbing at foods

Crying when food stops or the bowl is empty

THE SIGNALS THAT YOUR BABY WANTS LESS FOOD INCLUDE:

Turning their head away

Crying during the mealtime

Pushing food or bowl away with their hands

Clamping their mouth shut

Verbally informing you that they don't want the food

A great concept that often helps to make it clear when it comes to portion sizes for babies is based on work by Ellyn Satter. This suggests that, as a parent, you decide what and how food is offered, but let your baby decide if and how much is to be eaten. It can really help to remember this when feeding baby at mealtimes – they are ultimately in control of how much they eat.

Moving through meals: 1–2–3

Always start weaning with just one meal initially. This is to offer a gradual movement on to solids, to allow little ones to get used to food and the process of eating. Eating can be quite a hard skill to master, and too much all at once may put them off, or be difficult for their tummies to digest.

The pace at which you'll need to move from one meal to two to three meals a day varies from one family to another. Some babies take to solids quickly and will be on three meals fairly soon after introducing solids. Other babies aren't that fussed, moving to three meals fairly slowly. Ideally, baby will be on three meals between around seven and nine months of age, to make sure they are getting plenty of practice with eating, getting used to mealtime routines and also getting plenty of nutrients into their diet. It's good to move up to another meal – breakfast, lunch or dinner – once your little one seems to have accepted the first meal and is gaining confidence in the whole process of eating. During my step-by-step 30-day guide (see page 76), it's up to you when you add in another meal. You can use the flowchart opposite to help you decide.

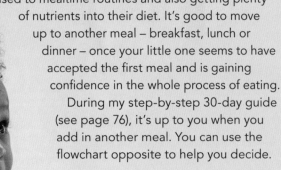
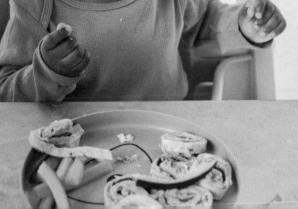

IS BABY ENJOYING CURRENT MEAL?

NO → Leave it a little longer before adding another.

YES ↓

IS BABY IN A NICE ROUTINE AROUND MEALTIMES AND SEEMS TO KNOW WHEN TO EXPECT THEM?

NO → Try to establish more of a routine before moving on to the next meal.

YES ↓

ARE THEY SWALLOWING MOST OF THE FOOD AT MEALTIMES?

NO → Are they baby-led weaning? It can take a little longer if so. Check baby is developmentally ready for solids and process to next step.

YES ↓

DO YOU FEEL READY TO OFFER A SECOND MEAL?

NO → Get yourself prepped: have a read through the 30-day guide and give it a little time.

YES ↓

GO FOR IT

Introducing allergens

Allergies is one of the areas of weaning and child nutrition that really makes parents nervous, which is completely understandable. It's all too easy to read horror stories online and most of us know friends or relatives who have children with allergies.

However, it's important to know that only around 5 percent of two-year-olds in the UK have a proven food allergy, and so the likelihood of your baby having an allergy is fairly low. Some babies will be allergic to foods before they are even introduced into their diet and some allergies can also develop later in life. In the UK, common foods which can cause allergies include:

* eggs
* peanuts
* tree nuts, such as almonds, cashew nuts and walnuts
* dairy foods, such as cow's milk, cheese and yoghurt
* fish and shellfish
* wheat, found in bread, couscous, pasta
* soya, such as soya milk and tofu (soya is also found in many breads)

These are the allergens most prominent in young children's diets. But there are actually 14 allergens that are required, by law, to be shown on food labels in the UK. These include the above, but also:

* mustard
* celery
* sulphur dioxide (found in dried foods such as dried apricots and used as a preservative in some manufactured foods)
* lupin (found commonly in baked goods)
* molluscs
* sesame (found in tahini and hummus)

In recent years, there has been a great deal of research looking into allergies in young children. Previously, advice was to delay the introduction of certain allergens when weaning. However, research from around the world, including two substantial studies from the UK (see page 207), has found that introducing allergenic foods at the same time as other solid foods may protect infants from developing a food allergy.

This has led to a change in advice in the UK as well as many other countries worldwide. The new advice suggests that we should:

Introduce allergens during weaning, along with other foods, from around six months.

Avoid delaying or excluding allergens (unless there is a known allergy) as this may actually increase the risk of a food allergy developing.

Aim to introduce the main allergens, especially eggs, peanuts and tree nuts (ground or as nut butters), pasteurised dairy foods, fish/seafood and wheat (as long as they are part of your family's diet) before 12 months of age, one at a time.

Continue to give these foods to your baby regularly as part of their usual diet (unless not tolerated) to help reduce the chances of an allergy developing later.

Encourage diversity in your baby's diet.

Some infants may be at higher risk of developing a food allergy, and this is likely to be the case if:

1. They have eczema, particularly early onset and moderate to severe eczema.

2. They already have a known food allergy.

Having a sibling or a parent with a food allergy isn't necessarily an indicator that a child is 'at risk' of developing a food allergy, but a specialist will take this into account along with the above indicators of a child being 'high risk'.

If you believe your little one to be 'high risk' of developing a food allergy, it's suggested that you may benefit from introducing egg and peanut allergens to your baby earlier than six months of age. However, this is beyond the scope of this book and I would recommend that you seek advice from a GP who is familiar with infant food allergies or a paediatric allergy specialist/dietitian as early as possible and preferably before you start offering solid foods to your baby. Don't worry if your little one is 6 months already, but it's important not to delay the introduction of allergenic foods beyond 12 months of age.

If your baby has an immediate reaction to any foods, it's important to stop giving the food, see a GP and ask for a referral to a specialist allergy clinic. In the case of severe symptoms (see opposite) dial 999 for urgent help.

SYMPTOMS OF AN ALLERGIC REACTION

IMMEDIATE-TYPE FOOD ALLERGY
*Typically happens within
30 minutes of eating food*

Symptoms:
* Swollen lips, face or eyes
* Itchy skin rash e.g. hives
* Abdominal pain, vomiting

Severe symptoms (very rare):
* Swollen tongue, persistent cough, hoarse cry
* Difficult or noisy breathing
* Pale or floppy, unresponsive/unconscious

What to do?
* If your baby has any severe symptoms (anaphylaxis), immediately dial 999 for help.
* Mild moderate symptoms are not dangerous. Dial 111 for advice.
* Avoid the causative food, do NOT reintroduce.
* Speak to your GP to discuss review by a specialist paediatric/allergy team.
* NICE recommends any baby with multiple food allergies or severe symptoms (anaphylaxis) should be referred to a hospital team.

**Reproduced courtesy of the BSACI
and the Food Allergy Group of the BDA**

DELAYED-TYPE FOOD ALLERGY
*Symptoms occur hours
after the food trigger*

Gut symptoms:
* Recurrent abdominal pain, worsening vomiting/reflux
* Food refusal or aversion
* Loose/frequent stools (more than 6–8 times a day)
* Constipation/infrequent stools (2 or less per week)

Skin symptoms:
* Skin reddening or itch over body
* Worsening eczema

What to do?
* Stop the suspected food; symptoms should resolve after a few days.
* If symptoms reoccur or are severe, or your child is not growing, then see your GP.
* NICE recommends that babies with any of the following should be referred to a specialist clinic:

    * Faltering growth
    * Reflux or gut symptoms resistant to treatment
    * Food refusal
    * Eczema which worsens with specific food

Delayed allergy cannot trigger anaphylaxis.

How to introduce allergens

Introducing allergens can make parents very nervous, so here is my step-by-step flow chart to help you introduce allergens to your baby safely:

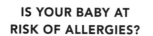

IS YOUR BABY AT RISK OF ALLERGIES?

NO → Follow the step-by-step guide opposite

YES

Seek advice as early as possible from someone who specialises in allergies, or your healthcare professional. It's important not to delay the introduction beyond 12 months of age

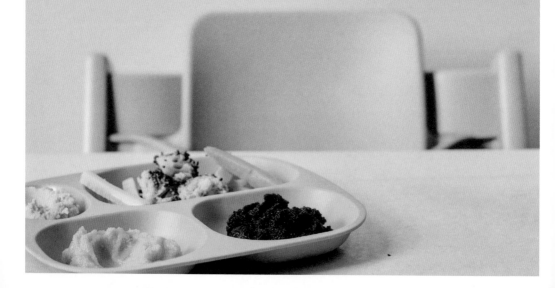

1	Introduce allergens as part of baby's normal diet when baby is ready for solid foods – aim to offer them before 12 months of age.
2	Only offer allergens to your baby when they are well.
3	Offer an allergen, starting with eggs ideally, as long as they are part of your family's diet.
4	Make sure the allergen is offered in an age-appropriate form to avoid risk of choking e.g. mashed egg, ground nuts or nut butters.
5	Offer the allergen early in the day the first few times so you have time to look out for a reaction.
6	Offer just a tiny amount of the allergen initially and don't offer any other new foods that day.
7	Be aware of the reactions you might be looking for (see page 59).
8	Leave two- or three-days' gap before offering a different allergenic food for the first time, so you can spot a delayed reaction. If a reaction occurs, stop giving the food and see your GP for a referral/advice.
9	Once introduced and tolerated, try to include the allergen regularly, as part of your little one's diet (e.g. at least once a week).
10	Offer peanut as the next allergen and follow the same steps 2–9 in order above.
11	Continue to offer other allergens (if eaten as part of your family's diet) in the same way as above, including tree nuts, cow's milk, wheat, seeds, fish, seafood and soya, and aim to introduce them all by around 12 months of age.

Foods to avoid

Once your little one is six months old, most foods are fine to add to their diets. Foods need to be served in an appropriate way (see choking hazards on page 46) for baby's age and stage, but luckily most foods we eat as adults, including all the foods in my 30-day guide and those in the recipes in this book, are fine to offer to babies and toddlers from six months.

The few foods that we should avoid giving to baby include:

Sugar and sugary foods are not recommended to be added to babies' foods and it's best to keep added sugar in babies' diet to a minimum. There is often sugar added into everyday foods such as bread, sauces and cereals. All forms of sugar, including foods and ingredients such as sweets, cakes, granulated sugar, honey, agave syrup and fruit juice, count as 'added' sugars. You can't avoid sugar completely (and you don't have to), but it's important to try to keep baby's intakes low.

Salt and salty foods aren't good for developing kidneys, and only a tiny amount of salt is needed in young children's diets. For this reason, it's good to avoid adding any salt to a baby's or toddler's meals and to try to keep salt intakes as low as possible. As with sugar, it's impossible to avoid salt completely – bread, crackers, sauces and cereals will all contain some added salt. Try to check labels and avoid adding it to a young child's food for as long as possible.

Honey isn't recommended until baby is one year of age, as it may contain bacteria that could be dangerous for an immature immune system. In babies over one year, honey should be fine from a bacterial point of view, but remember it's still an added sugar. Keep it to a minimum in children's diets.

Unpasteurised dairy hasn't been treated, which means it can contain bacteria which could be harmful. It's best to offer pasteurised, plain dairy products to babies and toddlers. Additionally, avoid offering mould-ripened soft cheeses and soft blue-veined cheese to babies and young children, as there's a higher risk that these cheeses might carry a bacteria called listeria. However, you can offer these to baby if they have been cooked in a recipe first.

Runny, soft-cooked eggs are fine to offer to baby if they have a Red Lion stamp on them (in the UK), which means the hens have been vaccinated for salmonella. If they aren't Red Lion-stamped, you can still offer eggs to your baby, just make sure they are cooked all the way through.

Raw fish, raw meat or undercooked shellfish are not recommended as foods for young babies simply because of the potential risk of food poisoning. A baby's immune system isn't as strong as an adult's, meaning they are more vulnerable to bugs and food poisoning.

Shark, swordfish or marlin can be high in mercury, which can affect your baby's developing nervous system and therefore should be avoided. It's also recommended in the UK that girls (of all ages) have no more than two portions of oily fish (e.g. salmon, mackerel, sardines) a week.

Rice milk can contain small amounts of arsenic and so is best avoided in large quantities. Rice milk isn't recommended until a child is five years of age. Rice is, however, fine to offer from around six months.

A few other foods aren't recommended for babies as they are potential choking hazards. For example, grapes and nuts shouldn't be offered whole until baby is five years of age. Whole nuts should be ground or offered as nut butters, and grapes should be quartered, lengthways. See page 47 for more on this.

Drinks

Water and baby's usual milk (see page 25) are the best drinks to offer to your baby and young toddler. Children don't need fruit juice, soft drinks or diluted squash to help keep them hydrated. Often when these drinks are offered, it can encourage children to reject water and many contain sugars that aren't good for baby's teeth.

Between 6 and 12 months, babies need only small sips of water with their meals (maybe more on hot days or when very active). Offering water at this point is more about getting them used to sipping fluids from an open cup and familiarising them with the taste of water. Formula-fed babies may need small amounts of water in very hot weather before six months of age, but it's recommended that this water is boiled first and then allowed to cool before offering it to baby. You don't need to boil and cool water for a baby over six months – water straight from the tap is fine.

AGE	TOTAL FLUID INTAKE RECOMMENDATIONS (FROM FOOD AND DRINK) (ML/DAY)	AS CUPS (A CUP IS AROUND 200ML)
Age 6–12 months	800–1000	Sips of water with meals
1–2 years	1100–1200	3–4 cups
2–3 years	1300	4–5 cups

Supplements for baby

For young babies in the UK there are certain supplements that are recommended to be offered daily. These include vitamins A, C and D.

Vitamin A and vitamin C are recommended for all babies from six months of age or from when baby is having less than 500ml of formula milk a day, right up until they are five years of age.

Vitamin D supplements are recommended from birth for a breastfed baby, or from whenever a baby is having less than 500ml of formula milk a day. This is simply because formula milk is already supplemented with vitamin D. The recommendation is for babies to have 8.5–10mcg a day under one year, and a 10mcg daily supplement after that, until they are five years of age.

You can get supplements that contain the right levels of vitamins A, C and D in one pack – the Government's Healthy Start Supplements are a good option – ask your local Health Visiting team for more information.

If your baby has allergies and is on a restricted diet, it's important to talk to your allergy specialist or dietitian to ensure they are getting all the nutrients they need from their current diet. In some cases, additional supplements (or fortified foods) might be necessary for your baby, so talk to your health visitor, GP or a registered nutritionist/dietitian as they can help you decide what your baby might need.

Having too many supplements can be harmful, so don't offer too many at the same time. Check the amounts recommended on the packet and avoid giving multiple supplements containing the same nutrients e.g. a baby multivitamin supplement plus a vitamin A supplement. Have a chat with a healthcare professional or pharmacist before offering more than one supplement to baby.

ESSENTIAL NUTRIENTS FOR WEANING

The macronutrients

These make up the building blocks of our diets and are needed in relatively large amounts from the foods we eat. Splitting foods into relevant food groups by their macronutrients can help simplify how to 'balance' out meals.

▼

CARBOHYDRATES

Carbohydrates are needed to provide energy to the body, which is especially essential for a baby growing at such a fast rate. They provide vitamins and minerals such as calcium, iron and B vitamins and are found in foods such as bread, potatoes, rice, pasta, cereals and grains (e.g. oats and bulgur wheat).

Fibre
is a part of many carbohydrate foods. Babies only need this in small amounts, as it can fill up tiny tummies in place of other foods. It's fine to include fibre (including wholegrains) in baby's diet, but it's best not to focus purely on wholegrains or high-fibre foods. From two years of age, you can start moving towards a diet that contains more wholegrains.

▼

PROTEINS

Protein is a macronutrient made up of amino acids, needed for growth, development and maintenance of health. Good sources of protein are found in beans, lentils, pulses, nut butters, meat, fish, dairy and eggs.

Many individual plant-based proteins don't contain the full range of essential amino acids that the body needs. If you're offering your baby a variety of protein foods, including lentils, beans, pulses and grains (grains also contain proteins) each day, it's unlikely to be a problem. Combining grains such as bread, pasta or rice, with pulses or beans helps to offer a range of all the essential amino acids. You don't always have to combine them at each meal, but a variety of grains and proteins throughout the day should help.

▼

FATS

There are different types of fat – it is recommended that we eat less saturated fat and more mono- and polyunsaturated fat. This is the same for babies too. Fats provide vital energy as well as help the body to absorb certain fat-soluble vitamins (vitamins A, D, E and K). Fats also have an important function as structural building blocks to our body cells. Found in oils, spreads, dairy foods, fish, nuts, seeds, meat and avocado. It's best to focus mainly on healthier fat options such as avocado, olive oil, oily fish, ground nuts and seeds.

▼

Omega-3

is a type of fatty acid needed for healthy brain and vision development and is found largely in oily fish, such as salmon, mackerel, sardines, trout and herring. This important fatty acid contributes to the normal functioning of the heart and brain development in infants. If your little one doesn't eat oily fish, then you can opt for other sources of omega-3 (many of which are plant-based), such as flaxseed oil or ground flaxseeds, ground walnuts, ground chia seeds or omega-3 enriched eggs.

In the UK, the advice for adults is to try to have two portions of fish a week, one of which should be oily. It's good to try to follow this advice for babies and infants too – just remember that babies need much smaller portions than adults.

ZINC

Zinc is essential for immune function and growth and repair of the body. It is found mainly in foods that also contain iron and protein (see page 66). Including a variety of these should ensure baby gets enough zinc too.

VITAMIN C

Vitamin C is abundant in fruits and vegetables including broccoli, dark green leafy vegetables, peppers, potatoes, tomatoes, kiwi fruit, oranges berries and mango. It is important for protecting the body's cells as well as supporting healthy skin and the immune system.

▲   ▲

The micronutrients

These are vitamins and minerals that are needed in varied and small amounts to help maintain overall health and support growth and development. Trying to calculate a baby's daily intake of each micronutrient would be impossible, so the best way to ensure that they get these important micronutrients is simply by offering a variety of foods each day from the main food groups (see page 114). However, some of these micronutrients are recommended to be supplemented in your baby's diet (see page 65).

▼   ▼

VITAMIN D

Vitamin D is needed alongside calcium for the normal growth and development of bones in children. Vitamin D helps the body to absorb calcium and helps to maintain muscle and bone function as well as having a role in the normal functioning of the immune system. Between April and September in the UK our main source of vitamin D comes from the sun, but babies aren't usually exposed to sunlight for any length of time. Food sources include oily fish, egg yolks, red meat and fortified foods and milks, but these alone don't provide enough and so supplements are recommended (see page 65).

VITAMIN A

Vitamin A (also known as retinol) contributes to immune function as well as normal vision and keeps the skin healthy. Beta-carotene is converted into vitamin A in the body and so including beta-carotene-rich foods also helps to provide vitamin A. Good sources include dairy foods, eggs and oily fish as well as fortified spreads. Beta-carotene is found in orange-coloured fruits and vegetables, such as carrots, apricots, sweet potatoes and butternut squash, and also dark green leafy vegetables, such as spinach.

IODINE

Our bodies use iodine to make thyroid hormones which are needed for normal bone and brain development in babies and young children, as well as growth in infancy. Dairy foods and white fish are the main sources of iodine in the UK diet. Some cereals and grains do contain iodine, but in variable amounts as it depends on when and where they are grown. If your little one doesn't eat fish or dairy foods it might be worth choosing iodine-fortified foods and/or a supplement (speak to your GP or health visitor about supplements). Some plant milks and dairy alternatives on the market fortify with iodine, but not all of them, so it's good to check labels.

IRON

Iron is needed for normal brain development in children, and helps to maintain a healthy immune system. Most of a baby's iron stores come from mum during pregnancy, and last around 4–6 months before they start to decline. From six months, after first tastes, iron-rich foods need to be included regularly in baby's diet. These include egg yolk, red meat, lentils, fortified cereals and beans. Try to include iron-rich foods early on in the weaning journey, after first tastes, and offer iron-rich foods at least a couple of times a day once mealtimes have been established. Iron is generally less well absorbed from plant-based sources such as beans, lentils, pulses, nut butters, hummus and dark green leafy vegetables. Vitamin C may help with the absorption of iron at a meal, so add foods such as broccoli, tomatoes, peppers and fresh fruits alongside iron-rich plant foods.

B VITAMINS

This group of vitamins includes thiamine, riboflavin, niacin, vitamin B6, vitamin B12 and folate. They are essential for helping release energy from food and keeping the immune system, nervous system and red blood cells functioning well. B vitamins are found in a wide variety of foods, including wholegrains, meat, dairy, fish and eggs. Vitamins B6 and B12 are harder to get in a plant-based diet. Choose fortified foods such as breakfast cereals and nutritional yeast, as well as beans, pulses, nuts and seeds to get a bit extra in your child's diet. If your little one doesn't eat any animal products, a vitamin B12 supplement or plenty of B12-fortified foods is likely to be necessary.

CALCIUM

Needed for normal growth and development of bones – important for a rapidly growing baby! Calcium also has a role in muscle function and cell division. In the UK diet, calcium largely comes from cow's milk and dairy foods, but it's also found in plenty of other foods such as dark green leafy vegetables, bread, tofu, ground nuts and seeds. If your little one doesn't eat dairy there are plenty of alternative sources of calcium, such as fortified plant milk, fortified cereals, calcium-set tofu, ground seeds and nuts, lentils and beans, bread and bread products, and dark green leafy vegetables. Calcium absorption is affected by other aspects of the diet, but as long as you are offering a variety of foods each day, your baby should be able to absorb enough calcium from these sources.

Vegetarian and vegan babies

Offering only plant foods, or plant foods and some dairy, might take a bit more planning to make sure you get the balance right for babies. It's always worth chatting about this with a healthcare professional (ideally a registered nutritionist/dietitian) before you begin weaning.

When it comes to milk, breastmilk is the best option for a vegan baby as there are currently no suitable vegan formulas available in the UK. Breastfeeding for as long as possible can also help to provide a substantial contribution to the nutrients that your baby will need throughout their first year and beyond.

As you start weaning your baby, make sure you offer a wide range of beans, pulses, grains and vegetables to ensure you're offering plenty of nutrients in baby's diet. It can be trickier to get the following nutrients in a vegan or vegetarian diet, so these will need more attention:

* protein   * omega-3

* fats   * vitamin B12

* iron   * calcium

* iodine

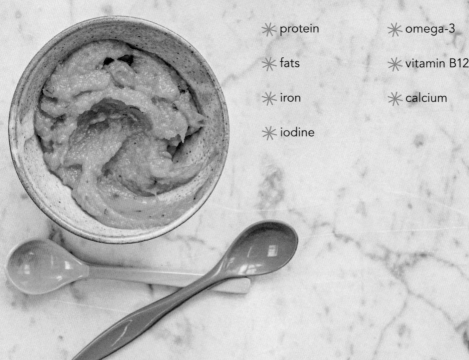

PREPPING FOR WEANING

Getting your equipment together

Basic kitchen equipment is all you need to start weaning – a knife, a chopping board, a bowl, a spoon and a pan. However, there are some things that you can add to these everyday basics to help make the whole process easier:

STEAMER

Can come in very handy, especially for prepping baby's first foods and veggies. You can always use a steaming basket or a colander over a pan of hot water if you don't have a steamer.

BLENDER

Useful if you want to offer purees. Blenders can be useful later on, too, for making sauces and curries, etc. You can use a mini hand blender, smoothie blender, or whatever gadget you already have at home. A fork can work just fine for many mashes!

PLASTIC OR BAMBOO PLATES, BOWLS AND UTENSILS

Really useful to minimise breakages early on, when cutlery, plates and cups often end up thrown on the floor as baby experiments and develops their skills around hand–eye coordination. Plastic or bamboo cutlery also don't conduct heat and so are better options at the start of weaning.

HIGH CHAIR

Ensure that baby can sit comfortably and nice and upright – not leaning back or slumped forward. It's ideal if they have a footrest to support their feet and allow them to keep their back straight when sitting. Removable trays are a good idea, as you can remove and bring the chair to the table so baby can sit with you.

BIBS, SPLASH MATS AND WASHABLE WIPES

For the mammoth clean-ups! Weaning is a messy time. These are necessary mainly for your sanity and for reducing your wash load!

POTS TO FREEZE, STORE AND CARRY FOOD

So many different pots are available! They don't have to be fancy, but go for ones that are reusable and can be frozen, as well as ones with lockable lids, to minimise spilling on the go. Ice-cube trays can be handy if you're making up purees in bulk, as well as reusable freezer bags to store frozen cubes of food.

OPEN CUPS

It's good to get baby used to sipping out of an open cup or beaker, rather than just a bottle or a valved cup when they first start solid foods. This can help them learn to eventually drink from a glass like an adult. I recommend offering an open cup alongside mealtimes with a small amount of water from the start of weaning.

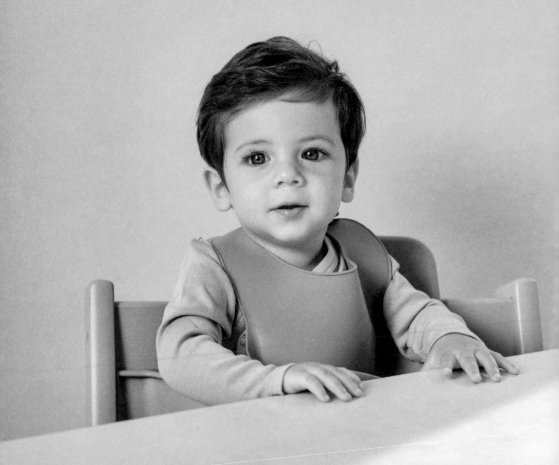

Cooking for your baby

STEAMING Steaming is great for cooking vegetables and fruits as it helps to preserve nutrients such as vitamin C and some B vitamins such as riboflavin.

BOILING If you aren't able to steam, try boiling vegetables in a small amount of water for as short a time as possible to get the texture you want. Some nutrients can leach out of foods into the water when boiling, so the less water the better; use cooking water for mashing, if needed. As baby gets more confident with textures you can cook for less time too, which retains more nutrients.

MICROWAVING You can use a microwave to cook baby's foods but be aware that microwaving can create hot spots, so be sure to stir baby's food well and allow it to cool right down before offering.

ROASTING Roasting vegetables and foods can result in harder textures than steaming or boiling. This is fine for later on when your baby is used to a variety of textures. You could try steaming and then roasting foods for baby, which helps to soften and then allows you to add in extra flavours with herbs and spices.

FRYING Try to use rapeseed or olive oil when frying and avoid re-frying any oils. Avoid offering baby lots of fried foods regularly.

BAKING This is always a good option when you've moved on to more family meals – for example you could try my Spinach and Cheddar Muffins (page 188), Cheese Biscuits (page 192) and Carrot Oat Bars (page 191).

Food hygiene, storing and reheating

A lot of food hygiene for baby's foods is common sense, but it can be nice to have a quick reminder, especially if you are now doing more food prep than usual.

GENERAL HYGIENE GUIDELINES

✳ Wash your hands before prepping food, and wash baby's hands thoroughly before mealtimes.

✳ Keep kitchen surfaces, cooking utensils, chopping boards, pots and pans clean.

✳ Wash all of baby's feeding equipment in hot soapy water after use. There is no need to sterilise after six months, except for baby's bottles.

✳ Wash ingredients before prepping them and remove any tough skins from raw fruits and vegetables.

✳ Keep raw meat and eggs separate from other foods in the fridge and while cooking.

PREPPING AND STORING BABY'S FOOD

Cook food until piping hot and then cool before serving to baby.

Offer food for baby in a separate bowl from the one you cooked in, and add more if baby is still hungry. Avoid keeping food that has been eaten or touched by your baby (e.g. if a spoon has gone in and out of the bowl and baby's mouth), as bacteria from baby will have transferred to the food.

Throw away any half-eaten foods but store untouched foods in the fridge for up to 24 hours. You can also freeze any untouched food. Don't reheat more than once.

If batch-cooking or storing leftovers, cool food as quickly as possible before putting in the fridge or freezer (always within an hour and a half). If refrigerated use within two days (one day for rice dishes). Don't reheat more than once.

If batch-cooking and freezing food, cool as quickly as possible and then pop into freezer trays or pots with a lid. You can transfer to labelled freezer bags if you like.

Defrost frozen foods first in the microwave or by leaving in the fridge overnight. Reheat until piping hot and then allow to cool. Do not reheat more than once.

When offering water to a baby before six months, boil and cool the water first. Once baby is six months old, water can be offered straight from the tap.

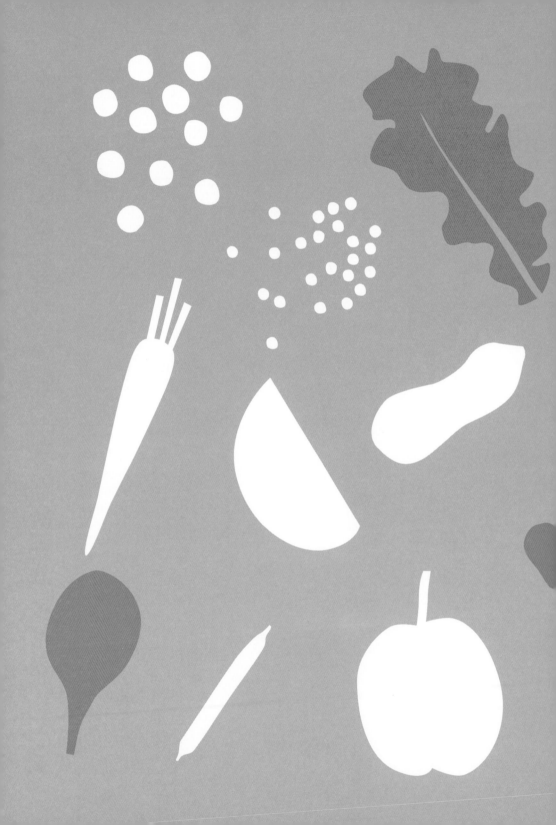

THE FIRST 30 DAYS

A STEP-BY-STEP GUIDE

2

This section will talk you through how to approach the first 30 days of your weaning journey, but please don't feel you have to follow these guidelines to the letter. They are just that – guidelines – to help you feel more confident about offering the first tastes of foods to your baby.

I'll walk you through each day, step-by-step, offering advice on textures, allergens and including iron-rich foods. I'll also show when to start combining ingredients, adding in some herbs and spices, and how much variety is ideal in the early days.

My approach to weaning starts with veggies, and then brings in plenty of variety and new ingredients alongside yet more veggies! The idea is to vary the savoury tastes that your little one is exposed to throughout their entire food experience; there is more to life than just apple!

If you don't have any of the vegetables I recommend throughout the 30-day guide, don't worry at all; just substitute some different veggies in their place or just use what you are eating as a family. These are not hard and fast rules.

Remember it's only tiny tastes of each vegetable initially. A new vegetable each day is ideal, but not essential; just aim for a variety.

Eat together...

When you follow the guide, if you can also make the vegetables part of your own meal and eat them alongside your baby, it can make weaning that much easier and help baby to accept foods more readily. Have the veggies on your plate and happily munch along or make a meal out of them for the whole family, such as a veggie pasta dish with broccoli pieces; a stew with kale or spinach; or some avocado on toast, so that you're sharing the same food as your little one at similar times.

A NOTE ON PORTION SIZES

I've included suggested portions for each recipe in this guide but these are likely to vary a lot depending on cooking styles, equipment used and how much milk or liquid is added. Try not to worry too much about portion sizes for baby. Some children eat a lot at the start of weaning while others eat very little, and the amount your baby will want to eat may vary from day to day too (see page 49). As a result of this, some of the recipes throughout this guide will provide surplus, which means you may have some leftovers to either eat yourself or to store in the fridge or freezer for a later date.

BABY'S USUAL MILK

In the recipe suggestions that follow, I mention 'baby's usual milk' can be added to some recipes. It's best to use baby's usual milk initially, such as breast milk or formula, as baby is familiar with it, and this can help encourage acceptance of these new tastes. After the first few food attempts, you can use full-fat cow's milk instead, if you prefer. Remember, though, cow's milk is one of the main allergens (see page 56). If your baby has been drinking formula milk with no problems they are likely to tolerate dairy products well. For breastfed babies this may be their first exposure to cow's milk so treat it as a new allergen (see page 60).

Freezing leftovers

Untouched leftovers – whether finger foods or purees – can be added to ice-cube trays/freezer bags and frozen for use later. Remember not to reheat anything more than once (see page 75). Bear in mind that the puree stage is very short, so you don't need huge amounts of frozen purees from the early days of weaning.

MYTH BUST!
—
'I should delay giving my baby green leafy vegetables'

Some countries recommend leaving foods such as spinach, chard and other dark green leafy vegetables until later on in the weaning journey, as they can be high in nitrites. You can leave these until later if you prefer, but that isn't the guidance in the UK and the amount of these foods that baby is likely to eat will be minimal and therefore nowhere near the limits for 'safe levels'.

Days 1–10
Shopping list for the first 10 days

You will only need a tiny amount of each of these, so just buy as part of your usual shopping or buy one extra, and eat up the leftovers yourself. Don't forget to complete the notes page (page 87).

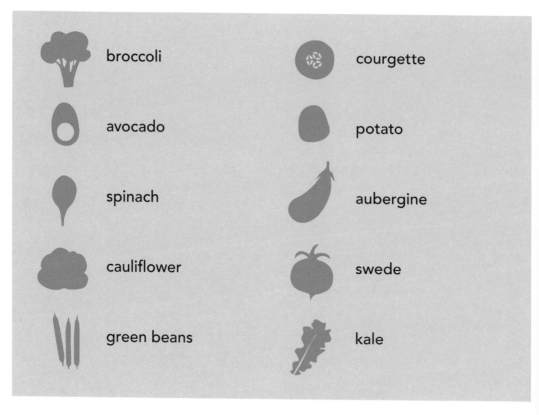

broccoli	courgette
avocado	potato
spinach	aubergine
cauliflower	swede
green beans	kale

Wash your veggies

Remember to wash all foods for baby before prepping them and remove tough skins from raw fruits and vegetables (see page 74).

BEFORE YOU BEGIN ON DAY 1:

○ Get the equipment you need for weaning (see page 71).

○ Buy all the ingredients you need so you're ready to go.

○ Plan your own meals so you can include the veggies below in your own dinner where possible.

○ Make sure baby is well and you've chosen the perfect time of day (see page 48).

Remember that this is all about tiny tastes and repeated exposures. We're not expecting baby to eat and appreciate all of the foods you're offering at these very first meals. One or two spoons might be all they manage, if that, and that's perfectly fine too.

TYPICAL MEAL PLAN AT SIX MONTHS OLD

This is a very general guide to show you how your little one's first meal might fit in around milk feeds but all babies will have a different routine. You will see that you will start with just one meal initially (see page 54 for more).

TIME OF DAY	FOOD
Morning	Baby's usual milk breast/bottle
Breakfast	
Nap time	Baby's usual milk breast/bottle before nap
Lunch	Veg puree and finger food
Nap time	Baby's usual milk breast/bottle before nap
Dinner	
Before bed	Baby's usual milk breast/bottle

DAY 1

Broccoli

Broccoli is a firm favourite of mine as a first food because it is just so different to anything baby has had before. It's also readily available – fresh or frozen – doesn't take long to prep or puree and is a great way of getting those savoury and slightly bitter notes on to baby's taste buds.

Makes around 2 portions

1. Boil or steam 75g broccoli (around 4 florets) for 8–10 minutes.
2. Once cooked, drain and remove one floret before blending the rest with a little of baby's usual milk until you get a texture you're comfortable with (see page 36). Alternatively, you can simply mash the broccoli up really well with a fork and a little cooking water or your baby's usual milk if you think baby is ready for thicker textures.
3. Serve a couple of teaspoons of the puree with the remaining floret of broccoli.

—

Broccoli is great for little hands to hold the stalk and munch off the top.

TIP

For this first week or so, offer one or two teaspoons of food to baby as a guide, along with a finger food stick or two. Offer more if baby wants more, or freeze any leftovers.

DAY 2

Courgette

Courgette is another fab first food as it's fairly bitter but can be a little creamy at the same time. It is super-watery compared to broccoli, so you may need to add less (if any) extra fluid. However, you can still add a little of baby's usual milk for a familiar taste if you prefer.

✳ Removing the skin is optional when blending, but for the first few times offering it as a finger food it's good to remove it as it can be a little hard for baby to chew.

Makes 1–2 portions

1. Cut 120g courgette into sticks the size and shape of an adult finger. Remove the skin from some of the sticks and boil or steam for about 5 minutes.
2. Remove a couple of the skinless sticks to serve as finger foods and blend or mash the rest.
3. Serve a couple of teaspoons of the puree/ mash with the remaining sticks of courgette.

—

Finger foods that you can easily squash between your finger and thumb are ideal, so check the texture of the courgette sticks are just right for baby before serving.

TIP

Don't worry if your baby doesn't take to any of the foods you're offering right away. That's completely normal. Just get the camera out for those unsightly facials!

DAY 3

Avocado

Avocado is a great way to add a totally different texture to your baby's repertoire. It is a great source of healthy fats as well as B vitamins and minerals. Using avocado is a quick option too, as it doesn't need cooking and works well as a finger food, as long as you have a ripe avocado.

✳ Leaving the skin on the bottom half of the avocado makes it easier for baby to hold.

Makes 1–2 portions

1. Slice ½ an avocado lengthways and remove one stick (roughly the size and shape of an adult finger) with the skin on. Carefully remove the skin from the top half of the avocado finger, leaving the bottom part on.
2. Scoop the rest of the avocado half out, removing the stone, and mash it up really well with some of baby's usual milk.
3. Offer the mash to baby on a spoon alongside the avocado finger.

—

Avocado doesn't freeze well, so it's probably a good one to eat on the day. Why not try the Guacamole recipe on page 171.

TIP

Raw foods are fine to offer to a baby, as long as they have soft textures. Cucumber jelly (the inside bits) and avocado work well as first finger foods. Remove any tough skins and only offer them if you can squidge them nicely between your finger and thumb.

DAY 4

Potato

Potatoes have a neutral taste, so you can easily add them to other ingredients such as kale without stealing the show when it comes to the flavour.

✳ Remove the skin of the potatoes initially, as they are a little tough to cope with without the munching or chewing skills that baby will develop later.
✳ This recipe makes a few portions – you can either have some mash yourself, or freeze any leftovers.

Makes 3–4 portions

1. Peel the skin from 1 medium baking potato (about 200g) and chop it into sticks roughly the size and shape of an adult finger.
2. Boil or steam the potato sticks for 10–12 minutes, until fairly soft.
3. Once cooled, remove half of the sticks and mash the other half really well with a potato masher, adding a splash or two of baby's usual milk and/or some cooking water to loosen.
4. Serve a few spoonfuls of the potato mash alongside a couple of sticks of potato fingers.

TIP

Quite a few of the recipes (e.g. spinach, kale, aubergine) suggest including some potato fingers as dippers, so if you can prep some sticks now, it may save you time later on.

DAY 5

Spinach

Spinach is perfect to offer your little one as it's a bitter and totally new taste. You can combine this with some leftover potato from yesterday and stir it together with a little of baby's usual milk. This can help thicken up the texture while still allowing those bitter notes to come through.

✳ Spinach is tricky to offer as a finger food at this age. If you want to offer it as a finger food, I'd suggest offering some potato sticks and simply dipping the potato in the puree for baby to self-feed.

Makes 1–2 portions

1. Steam 1 large handful of spinach (about 30g) for about 2 minutes or until wilted.
2. Blend until it makes a thin puree and add a splash of baby's usual milk.
3. Offer a couple of spoonfuls of puree in a bowl alongside a stick or two of potato from yesterday.
—
Spinach can be very different to what your little one has tasted before – it's much more bitter – so don't be surprised if they don't ask for more and pull a very unappreciative face. They are simply experiencing the unknown.

TIP
Don't worry in the slightest if nothing gets swallowed in these first days and weeks… it's all normal and baby will be playing and exploring at this stage.

DAY 6

Aubergine

Aubergine has a really nice neutral flavour, but it can be a funny texture for babies which is possibly why it's often left out of weaning recipes and your baby may show some surprise! However, aubergine is a favourite in my house and can help to add a very different texture to baby's repertoire.

✳ Try to use the other aubergine half for your own food today (see my Quick Quesadillas on page 142).

Makes 2–3 portions

1. Cut an aubergine in half lengthways. Bake one half in the oven at 200°C for 30–40 minutes, until the inside is soft and the skin peels away from the flesh.
2. Once cooked, leave the aubergine to cool a little and then scoop out the insides and discard the skin. Blend or mash really well and add a few splashes of baby's usual milk, if needed.
3. Serve with a spoon and offer another veg stick such as a potato finger or a stick of broccoli as a dipper.

—

Aubergine is great to add flavours to – yoghurt, lemon, paprika and tomato all go so well with aubergine and it's one of my favourite veggies to use in cooking.

TIP
If baby isn't trying finger foods and they are ending up on the floor, make sure you're demonstrating how to eat them by picking up a floret and eating it yourself.

DAY 7
Cauliflower

Cauliflower might be one to skip for very windy babies, but otherwise, it's a good one to explore as it has a very distinctive taste. It's super-easy to cook and mash and add to meals, and helps to bulk dishes out with fibre and nutrients.

Windy vegetables

If you find your baby becomes windy after tasting cauliflower, or any veg, don't worry, it won't cause harm – just reduce the number of windy foods you offer and gradually add them in small amounts at a later date. Remember this is about tiny tastes, not eating huge amounts of any food, including cauliflower. Some of the most 'windy' culprits include:

- ✳ brussels sprouts
- ✳ kale
- ✳ broccoli
- ✳ cabbage
- ✳ leeks
- ✳ onions

Makes about 2 portions

1. Boil or steam 85g cauliflower (about 3 florets) for 8–10 minutes. Take out all but one floret.
2. Blend the rest of the cauliflower and then add a little of baby's usual milk to loosen, if needed.
3. Offer the puree on a spoon together with the remaining cauliflower floret.

DAY 8
Swede

This is another ingredient that is easy to add to foods and dishes to bulk them out, just like potato. Remove the tough skin, then mash it up or offer it as soft sticks of finger food for baby to munch on just like other veggies.

✳ Try making some swede into a mash to go alongside your own food today so you don't end up wasting what's left. You can also freeze any leftovers in ice-cube trays or as sticks and use as fillers for other purees where needed.

Makes 1–2 portions

1. Remove the skin from 100g swede and chop into sticks the size and shape of an adult finger. Boil or steam for 12–15 minutes, until softened.
2. Remove a couple of sticks and mash or blend the rest, adding a little of baby's usual milk or some cooking water.
3. Serve the puree/mash alongside the sticks of swede.

TIP
Using cooking water or baby's usual milk helps to add extra nutrients to the purees or mashes you're making for baby.

DAY 9
Green beans

Green beans are a great food for the start of weaning. If you're offering them whole, cook them so they are nice and squidgy, but don't expect much to go in. This first stage is just about baby experimenting and learning some hand–eye coordination skills.

✳ Green beans are hard to mash, so you might need the blender for this one.

Makes about 1 portion

1. Top and tail 50g green beans, and remove any tough stringy bits. Steam or boil the beans for 10–12 minutes.
2. Take a few single green beans out for use as finger foods and blend the rest – add a little of baby's usual milk or some cooking water, if needed.
3. Serve the green bean puree on a spoon with a couple of green beans as finger foods.

TIP
Don't worry if the frequency or nature of your baby's poo starts to change during weaning. This can happen as they are adjusting to a brand-new diet. Keep an eye on it and see your health visitor if you're ever worried. Baby can go for some days without pooing, and that can be normal.

DAY 10
Kale

This is another brilliant one for introducing baby to bitter tastes. It's a fab way to expose baby to something totally new. However, kale can be a little grainy and tough to break down, so you might want to introduce kale mixed with potato or swede mash.

✳ Kale, as with spinach, is not great as a finger food early on. Try using a stick of swede or potato as a dipper for kale puree.
✳ Have something yourself that includes kale so your little one can see you enjoying it. Try my Mac and Cheese with Kale and Cauliflower (see page 152).

Makes 1–2 portions

1. Remove the stalks from about 30g (1 large handful) of kale and discard. Steam the leaves for 5–7 minutes, until wilted.
2. Blend the leaves with baby's usual milk or some of the cooking water until you get a fairly smooth puree. Kale may take a bit of extra blending (and a good blender!) as it's very fibrous and you may need to add some extra water or milk.
3. Serve the kale puree with a vegetable dipper.

TIP
Getting bitter tastes into baby's diet is a good idea early on so they can start building some familiarity with them. It can take 10 attempts before baby is more accepting of some foods, so keep offering all these veggies to baby as your weaning journey progresses (see page 34).

Notes

Make a note of what your baby enjoyed over the last 10 days.

Were there any foods that baby refused completely?
(Try these ones again soon!)

How did baby react to different tastes?

What did you expect for your first days of weaning and
what was the reality?

The next 10 days will continue to use the veggies we've already offered, as well as introducing some new foods. We'll also be experimenting more, combining ingredients and, as long as baby is around six months, adding in some allergens and iron-rich foods. As you move through the next 10 days of weaning, the meals will start to get more complex, so brace yourself for needing to spend a little more time cooking as baby works on their skills around eating.

ADDING MORE MEALS

If you feel that weaning is going well and baby is starting to accept food and seems really ready, you might want to move baby on to two meals a day over the next few days. Remember all babies are different – some may not be ready for another meal just yet while others can't wait to get going (check out page 54 to see if your little one is ready for more). Just remember that baby's milk is still important, so offer similar amounts to what you were offering prior to weaning.

Keeping things consistent

If you're continuing with just one meal a day then offer it at a similar time each day. When you do decide to move up to two meals, choose a time of day which works for you and continue to offer the second meal at around that time each day too. If you're adding in a new meal, stick to similar ingredients for both meals that are included in the 11–20-day guide, or just double up on the portion sizes and offer the second meal the next day. These are just ideas to give you inspiration and they don't need to be followed to the letter; you can swap cod for salmon, spinach for kale or try beans instead of lentils – whatever works for you. Just remember to offer new foods gradually, and follow the important steps when offering allergens (see page 56).

UPPING THE TEXTURES

If you've only offered purees so far, think about making the textures slightly more challenging. Add a little less liquid or simply mash or blend the ingredients a little less.

I've generally referred to mashing foods during the next 10 days, but you can still blend some of them if you prefer. Additionally, most meat and some veggies such as kale, green beans and red pepper don't mash well, so you will need to keep that blender out.

FINGER FOODS

If you haven't yet tried finger foods, give them a go in the next 10 days. Start with super-soft finger foods, and build your and baby's confidence at exploring them. Refer back to the choking section on page 44 if you're worried about this.

Some babies really take to finger foods and seem to prefer self-feeding in this way. If this is the case, keep offering both the spoon and finger food options at mealtimes, but you might want to try offering more variety of finger foods at mealtimes. You can always offer extra veggie sticks or use some of the tips included in the recipes to focus more on finger food options.

On the next page is a shopping list guide with the foods you'll need over the next 10 days. You can easily swap out fresh for some frozen, pre-cooked, dried or tinned options, but please be aware it may alter cooking times needed.

Days 11–20
Shopping list for the next 10 days

It's so important to add variety into your baby's diet early on – remember my five key principles (see page 12) – which is why I've included plenty over the next 10 days. It doesn't have to be exactly this list, and you can use veg you have already at home instead

Don't forget to complete the notes page (see page 97).

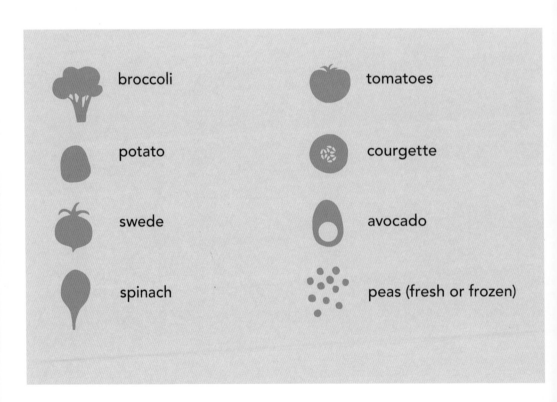

broccoli

tomatoes

potato

courgette

swede

avocado

spinach

peas (fresh or frozen)

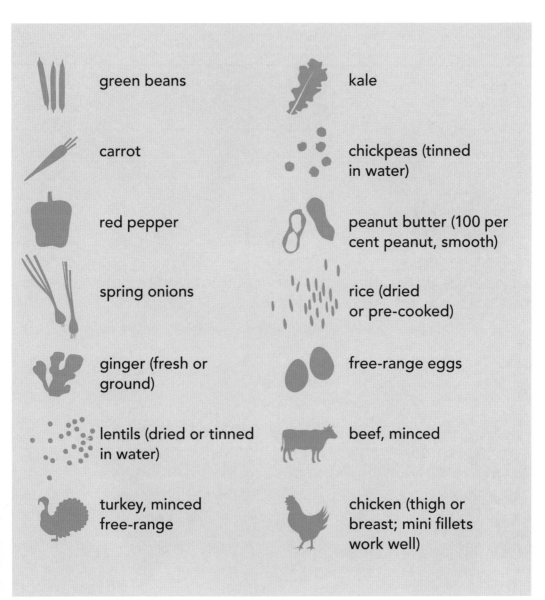

green beans

kale

carrot

chickpeas (tinned in water)

red pepper

peanut butter (100 per cent peanut, smooth)

spring onions

rice (dried or pre-cooked)

ginger (fresh or ground)

free-range eggs

lentils (dried or tinned in water)

beef, minced

turkey, minced free-range

chicken (thigh or breast; mini fillets work well)

DAY 11

Broccoli and potato

Combining ingredients is a good way to start building your confidence to make 'mini meals' for baby. It also offers baby more variety and repeat exposures to some of the veggies you've already tried. If you have frozen broccoli or potato left over from days 1–10, simply defrost, mix together, cook and serve these to baby instead.

✳ Potato doesn't always blend well as it's quite tacky; it's best to mash it instead. If the texture is still too thick, try adding some cooking water or baby's usual milk.

Makes about 1 portion

1. Peel and chop 50g potato into sticks the size and shape of an adult finger. Place in a steamer and cook for about 2 minutes.
2. Then add about 30g (2 florets) of broccoli to the steamer and cook for a further 10 minutes.
3. Take out one floret of broccoli and a couple of sticks of potato and mash the rest together really well, adding cooking water or baby's usual milk, if needed.
4. Serve the finger foods together with the potato and broccoli mash.

MAKING FINGER BALLS

To offer more finger food variety, you can turn many of these recipe ideas into balls. Mash the cooked ingredients together and roll into little balls, then bake them in the oven for 20 minutes at 200°C. This makes the balls a little more structured and easier for baby to hold.

DAY 12

Swede and lentils

Lentils are a great food for baby as they are nutrient-rich and a good source of iron. As they are quite high-fibre foods which young babies won't be used to, offer small amounts and gradually build on the amounts you're offering over time.

✳ For this recipe it's ideal if you can cook a batch of lentils for the whole family and set aside a couple of teaspoons for baby.
✳ I like to use ready-cooked lentils such as red, green and puy lentils in my cooking, but any will do for this recipe – just check there is no added salt or sugar.

TIP

Adding a little of baby's usual milk or some cooking water when mashing adds extra nutrients to baby's meals. Adding in extra calories and nutrients where you can is always a bonus.

Makes about 2 portions

1. Peel and chop 100g swede into finger-shaped sticks and steam for 12–15 minutes, until soft.
2. Meanwhile, cook 2 heaped teaspoons of lentils as per the packet instructions. If using pre-cooked, there is no need to cook or heat through.
3. Once cooked, drain and remove a few sticks of swede to serve as finger foods. Mash the rest of the swede really well with the cooked lentils, using a little cooking water or baby's usual milk, if needed.
4. Serve the mash with a few swede fingers.

DAY 13

Spinach and egg

Today we're trying our first new allergen – egg. Start with just a very small amount of any allergen initially, and build on this as you offer it more regularly. Make sure you've already read about the signs and symptoms of an allergic reaction on page 59, as well as details on how to introduce allergens, before you begin today's recipe.

※ This recipe requires some potato fingers to use as dippers, so if you have some in the freezer, defrost them in the microwave or overnight in the fridge, or see page 83 for how to make them.

※ If your little one reacts to egg, stop giving the food, don't offer it again and book to see your GP.

Makes about 1 portion

1. Steam 1 handful of spinach (about 30g) for about 2 minutes or until wilted.
2. Blend for a few seconds to make a puree.
3. Boil 1 free-range egg for 10 minutes. Make sure the egg yolk is well cooked, all the way through, as this is baby's first try. Remove the shell, once cooled.
4. Mash ½ of the egg really well and add a tiny amount (no more than about ½ teaspoon) to the spinach puree, mixing well.
5. Serve the spinach and egg mix along with a couple of potato fingers to use as dippers.

DAY 14

Green beans and chicken

It's good to get babies trying and tasting meat early on if you eat it as a family. This is to ensure it is more readily accepted and becomes a normal part of their diet. Meat can be a good source protein, B vitamins and iron. If you don't eat meat you could use butter beans, tofu or chickpeas here instead of chicken.

※ If your baby has been enjoying finger foods, you can simply offer a few green beans and a couple of sticks of well-cooked, soft chicken that squidges easily between your finger and thumb.

Makes about 2 portions

1. Wrap about 50g chicken fillets (breast or thigh) in foil and roast in the oven at 200°C for about 20 minutes.
2. Meanwhile, top and tail 50g green beans and remove any stringy bits. Steam for 10–12 minutes. Once ready, remove a few beans to offer as finger foods and leave to one side.
3. Once the chicken is cooked, remove a few thin strips of chicken to serve as finger foods and chop the rest into small pieces.
4. Add the chopped chicken to a blender along with the green beans. Blend to the desired consistency (you can't easily mash this one), adding a little of the green bean cooking water or baby's usual milk to make it a little smoother.
5. Serve the mash alongside the whole green beans and chicken fingers.

Tomatoes and chickpeas

This recipe doesn't really work as a finger food so add a side of veggie sticks as a dipper and show baby how to start dipping and scooping.

✳ Depending on the type of tomatoes you use, you might want to remove the skin if it's a little tough. Blending them skin-on is usually fine, but if you like, steam the tomatoes, let them cool and gently peel off the skin.

✳ This recipe doesn't need any extra fluid as the tomato adds plenty of water.

TIP

Tomatoes, acidic fruits and some berries can sometimes cause baby to have mild rashes around the mouth after eating them; this isn't usually an allergy, just an irritation of the skin. If you're worried check with your GP, but you can try spreading a little barrier cream around baby's mouth before offering these foods again.

Makes about 1–2 portions

1. Drain and rinse 30g pre-cooked chickpeas. Put the chickpeas in a steamer with 50g tomatoes and cook for about 5 minutes.
2. Blend the ingredients together for just a few seconds, so there is still a bit of texture left (these ingredients don't mash so well). Remove any whole pieces of tomato skin left in the mixture.
3. Serve with a stick of a cooked vegetable (such as broccoli) as a finger food dipper.

Courgette and beef

Beef is a great source of iron, so if it's part of your family's diet, include it early on to allow baby to become familiar with the taste.

✳ Sometimes babies are unsure of the texture of meat at first, so try offering it in different ways – pureed, minced with other foods, or as meatballs.

✳ If your little one doesn't take to meat, remember that foods such as ground nuts, lentils, chickpeas and beans can act as good replacements nutrient-wise.

Makes about 2 portions

1. Cut 100g courgette into finger-shaped sticks and remove the skin from a few of them. Steam the courgette sticks for 5 minutes. Remove the peeled sticks to offer as finger foods
2. Add 50g good-quality beef mince to a pan, with a little olive oil if needed, and cook for about 5 minutes over a medium heat, until browned all the way through.
3. Once cooked, add the mince to the rest of the courgette sticks and blend lightly for a few seconds to allow for some texture to remain.
4. Serve the beef and courgette mixture with the sticks of courgette.

MAKING FINGER BALLS

Meatballs are ideal for baby-led weaning. Mix 100g mince with 50g grated courgette and form into little balls. Bake in the oven at 200°C for about 20 minutes, turning halfway to make sure the mince is browned all the way through.

DAY 17

Avocado and peanut butter

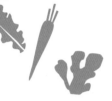

We are going to add another allergen today – peanuts. Nut butters are a great way to experiment a little with allergens, especially as there is so much variety out there. Cashew, almond and peanut butter are all staples in our house but go for 100 per cent nut varieties for babies.

* Check the advice on introducing allergens and the signs and symptoms to look out for before offering them to your baby each time (see page 56).
* If your little one reacts to the nut butter, stop offering it, don't offer it again, and book to see your GP.

Makes about 2 portions

1. Cut ½ an avocado into sticks for finger food – you can leave the skin on the bottom half for baby to grip. Scoop out the rest of the avocado and mash it up well.
2. Stir ½ teaspoon of peanut butter into a splash of boiled water or mix it with some of baby's usual milk, to loosen it.
3. Mix the peanut butter water into the avocado mash, stir well and serve along with a couple of avocado sticks.

TIP
If this meal is too small for your little one, or your little one prefers more finger foods at this stage, try offering more avocado sticks, or some fingers of food that baby has already had in their diet, such as broccoli or potato fingers.

DAY 18

Kale, carrot and ginger

This is a really delicious and refreshing option for baby and a great way of starting to experiment with flavours. Kale and carrot go so nicely with ginger. Why not make yourself a juice or smoothie with these ingredients to have too?

* Starting to experiment with flavours in baby's diet makes weaning super-exciting. It also helps to add new tastes to baby's palate, which helps to build familiarity with a real variety of foods.

Makes 1–2 portions

1. Remove the tough stalks from 1 small handful of kale. Steam the leaves for 5–7 minutes. Blend with a splash of cooking water or a little of baby's usual milk.
2. Meanwhile, peel 1 carrot and cut into sticks. Steam for about 10 minutes, until soft enough to squidge between your finger and thumb. Set aside a few sticks to offer as finger foods.
3. Mash the rest of the carrots with the kale puree and a tiny pinch of ground ginger (or a tiny grating of fresh).
4. Serve the mash to baby with the carrot sticks.

TIP
If your little one is wanting to grab the spoon, go ahead and let them. You can try having one spoon for you and one for them.

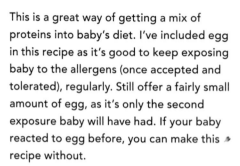

DAY 19

Peas, egg and rice

This is a great way of getting a mix of proteins into baby's diet. I've included egg in this recipe as it's good to keep exposing baby to the allergens (once accepted and tolerated), regularly. Still offer a fairly small amount of egg, as it's only the second exposure baby will have had. If your baby reacted to egg before, you can make this recipe without.

＊ Peas are a nutrition powerhouse, with plenty of vitamin C and protein.

Makes about 2 portions

1. Cook 25g white or brown plain rice as per the packet instructions. This might work better if you're having rice yourself today – make up a batch of rice for the family and take out about 50g cooked rice for baby.
2. Boil 1 free-range egg for 10 minutes. Make sure the egg yolk is well cooked. Remove the shell, once cooled. Mash the egg.
3. Meanwhile, steam or boil 20g frozen or fresh peas for 5 minutes.
4. Mix the peas, rice and 1 teaspoon of egg together and mash the mixture (or pop in a blender for a few seconds). Roll part (or all, if you prefer) of the mixture into a small ball to offer to baby as a finger food.
5. Mash the rest of the mixture further, adding a little cooking water, if needed.
6. Serve the rice and pea mash with a rice and pea ball.

DAY 20

Red pepper, turkey and spring onion

Turkey is a good food to experiment with if you eat it as a family, but you can always swap it for other meats such as chicken or beef, if you prefer. Turkey is a good source of protein and B vitamins, including vitamin B12. Chickpeas are a good vegetarian alternative for this recipe.

Makes 2 portions

1. Cut ½ red pepper into sticks, and remove any seeds. Steam for 8–10 minutes. Leave to cool for a minute and then gently peel off the skin.
2. Finely dice the white part of 1 small spring onion. Add to a pan with 50g turkey mince and a tiny bit of oil. Cook for about 5 minutes, until the turkey mince is browned all the way through.
3. Blend the turkey mixture and some of the pepper together for a few seconds, allowing for some texture to remain (this one doesn't mash well).
4. Serve the remaining sticks of pepper with the turkey and red pepper mash.

MAKING FINGER BALLS

Mix together 50g turkey mince with a diced spring onion, and roll the ingredients into balls. Bake in the oven at 200°C for about 20 minutes, turning halfway to make sure the mince is browned all the way through. Serve with some pepper fingers or dip in a red pepper puree.

Notes

Make a note of what your baby enjoyed over the last 10 days.

Which foods did baby reject completely?
(Try these ones again soon!)

How did baby react to different tastes?

What food combinations did baby enjoy the most?

How is baby coping with different textures?

_____

_____

_____

_____

_____

_____

_____

_____

This next stage is all about really building on those mini meals, adding in a variety of proteins, more allergens and starting to play with the flavours you're including in baby's foods. It's about getting experimental, adding in some new ingredients, and starting to create balanced meals for your baby. At this stage we can also start building in some sweeter tastes too, such as sweeter veggies and fruits, while still continuing to offer plenty of savoury and bitter flavours.

ADDING MORE MEALS

If you haven't thought about a second meal yet, now might be a good time to decide whether baby is ready for meal number two. It's important to move through meals gradually, so don't rush it and try to follow baby's lead on when they are ready (see page 54 for guidance).

You can repeat the recipes from earlier on in the guide to create extra meals for baby. A few more ideas include:

✳ potatoes, beef and tomatoes

✳ carrot, rice and butter beans

✳ broccoli and sweet potato with chicken

✳ kale with rice, kidney beans and cumin

✳ butternut squash with quinoa and lentils

✳ aubergine, chickpeas and tomato with potato fingers

✳ swede, kale and peas

✳ spinach, rice and chicken

Mixing things up

Combining familiar foods with new foods may help with your baby's acceptance. You don't necessarily want to be masking bitter or unfamiliar flavours with sweet ones, but offering foods that your baby has already accepted with a brand-new one may help them to accept new ones too.

TEXTURES

As baby is almost a month into weaning, it's a good time to really experiment with those textures. If you're still on a thin puree start to thicken it up by blending less and adding less liquid or simply start to mash foods instead, where possible. Some of the ingredients, especially meat, rice and some tougher veggies, may still need blending to get an easy texture for baby to manage, but you can always blend for less time, or mash part of the meal and serve finger foods too.

FINGER FOODS

Finger foods can help babies get used to more textures, so keep offering a variety. You'll still need to cook veggies pretty well, but you might be able to steam them for a little less time as baby gets more confident with them.

If your baby has really taken to finger foods, and prefers these to purees, most of the meals and recipes that follow can be easily adapted, such as:

* Use veggie sticks as a dipper for any of the purees/mashed options.

* Spread a thick mash on top of veggie batons or, once introduced, bread or toast.

* Mix ingredients for a puree with cooked potato or grains such as rice and quinoa and roll them into mini balls – you can then cook in the oven at 200°C for about 20 minutes to help them keep their shape.

* Bake foods into mini muffins or patties.

PORTION SIZES

If you feel like baby is ready for more in the way of portions, you can always add a few extra finger foods to each mealtime by boiling up some extra veg or adding a side of something they've enjoyed previously. You can also try doubling the recipes as these are just general portion guidelines. Towards the end of the month your baby may still only take a few spoonfuls at each meal, or they may be finishing the bowl; either is perfectly normal. If you're worried, do have a chat with your health visitor.

TIP

Please don't be put off if your baby isn't taking much or doesn't seem to 'like' some of the foods on offer. We've been really experimental during this journey and your baby has tried so many new foods so they are still learning and adapting their taste buds. Keep offering foods, even if rejected.

MEAL COMPLEXITY

As we move through these next 10 days the meals get somewhat more complex as we are using multiple ingredients and starting to use other methods of cooking and preparing baby's foods. Building baby's meals into your own meal plans so that you don't have to prepare separate meals for baby can save you time on cooking.

Days 21–30
Shopping list for the next 10 days

You don't have to buy all the ingredients here if you prefer not to, you can sub in ones you have more regularly at home and use fresh, frozen and pre-cooked options where you have them too. This shopping list is just to give you ideas and inspiration for the days ahead.

Don't forget to complete the notes page (see page 111).

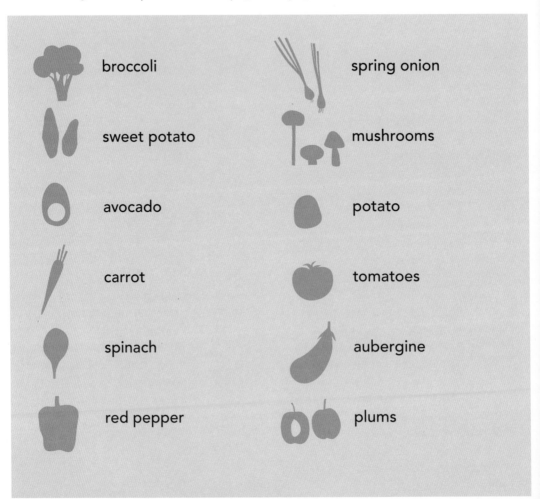

broccoli

sweet potato

avocado

carrot

spinach

red pepper

spring onion

mushrooms

potato

tomatoes

aubergine

plums

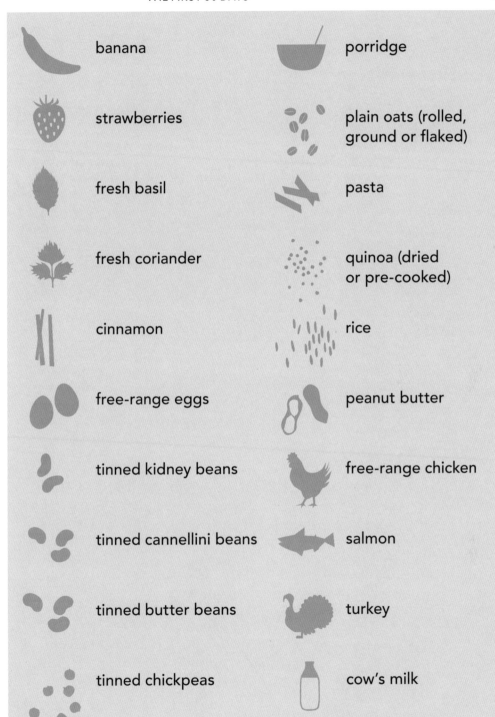

banana

strawberries

fresh basil

fresh coriander

cinnamon

free-range eggs

tinned kidney beans

tinned cannellini beans

tinned butter beans

tinned chickpeas

porridge

plain oats (rolled, ground or flaked)

pasta

quinoa (dried or pre-cooked)

rice

peanut butter

free-range chicken

salmon

turkey

cow's milk

DAY 21

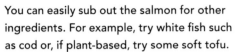

Broccoli, salmon and rice

You can easily sub out the salmon for other ingredients. For example, try white fish such as cod or, if plant-based, try some soft tofu.

Salmon is another allergen, so when offering it to baby for the first time, check back to page 56 for a reminder of how to introduce allergens safely.

* Salmon is a fab early food for your baby. It's a great source of omega-3 fatty acids for baby, and it's good to get them used to having fish early on.
* Your baby will only need a small portion of salmon, so include it in your own meal.
* If your little one reacts to the salmon, stop offering it, don't offer it again and book to see your GP.

Makes 1–2 portions

1. Wrap a piece of salmon in tin foil and bake in the oven at 200°C for about 20 minutes.
2. Meanwhile, cook about 15g rice as per the packet instructions. Alternatively, cook a batch of rice for yourself or your family and remove about 30g cooked rice for baby's meal.
3. Steam about 75g broccoli florets for 8–10 minutes (you can also add the broccoli to the rice while cooking for the last 8–10 minutes). Set aside 2 florets.
4. Once cooked, blend or mash 15g salmon with the cooked rice and the remaining broccoli florets until the ingredients are mixed but still have some texture left. When blending, add a little extra cooking water if needed.
4. Serve the mash with the broccoli florets.

DAY 22

Sweet potato, kidney beans and coriander

Sweet potato is a popular weaning food because it's easy to prepare, adds bulk to meals and is sweet, so babies tend to like it.

* Sweet potato is a good source of vitamin A, vitamin C and fibre.
* The kidney beans add protein to this dish. You will have some left over if you buy a tin of beans, so add to a stew, chilli or curry for your family.

Makes 2 portions

1. Peel 100g sweet potato and cut into sticks. Steam for about 10–12 minutes or until soft.
2. Meanwhile, drain and rinse 30g tinned kidney beans. Add them to the sweet potato after 5 minutes of steaming to heat through.
3. Once cooked, take out 2 or 3 sticks of the sweet potato and leave to one side.
4. Finely chop 1 small sprig of fresh coriander.
5. Mix the rest of the potato, the kidney beans and the coriander together and mash really well with a potato masher. Add a little cooking water if needed.
6. Serve the mash with the sticks of sweet potato.

MAKING FINGER BALLS

If your baby prefers finger foods simply roll the mash mixture into balls and offer to baby as they are, or bake in the oven at 200°C for about 20 minutes, to make them easier for baby to hold.

Avocado with chicken, quinoa and peanut butter dip

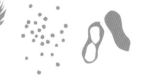

This is a delicious combination, and packed full of flavour and protein. The peanut butter is there just to make sure that, as long as baby has accepted and tolerated it the first time, we are offering the allergen fairly regularly in their diet. If your baby reacted to peanut butter before, you can easily leave it out.

* Using different grains, such as quinoa and barley, instead of just focusing on rice and pasta, can add a good dose of variety into baby's diet.
* If your family eats meat, offering chicken during the early weaning days can be helpful, and there are so many ways to serve it: soft strips of chicken, mashed/pureed chicken with veg, balls of chicken mince or shredded chicken, for example. If you're looking for a vegetarian option, try butter beans instead of the chicken.

Makes about 2 portions

1. Roast 1 small chicken breast or thigh (skinless) wrapped in tin foil in the oven at 200°C for 20–25 minutes, until tender but well cooked. Cut off one or two strips of chicken to offer as finger foods.
2. Meanwhile, cook about 15g quinoa as per the packet instructions, or use about 25g pre-cooked.
3. Cut an avocado in half, and cut out a slice as a finger food.
4. Destone and peel the rest of the avocado half and add to a blender with the cooked chicken and the quinoa.
5. Blend together the avocado, chicken and quinoa with ½–1 teaspoon of peanut butter until it all makes a nice mash. Add a little of baby's usual milk or cooking water, if needed.
6. Serve the mash with the strips of chicken and the avocado finger.

TIP

Once allergens are accepted without reaction, it's a good idea to offer them around once a week to ensure a tolerance is maintained.

MAKING FINGER BALLS

To make this into finger foods, simply keep the mash fairly thick and roll the mixture into little balls. Or offer avocado sticks rolled in a little pre-cooked quinoa alongside tender chicken strips with a peanut butter dip.

Spinach, strawberry and butter beans

This recipe is slightly fiddlier than the others so far, but it's totally worth it. Combining spinach and strawberry is a great way to get some bitter and sweet notes together in baby's meal. It's really experimental and surprisingly delicious – try a spinach and strawberry salad for yourself with a splash of balsamic vinegar! It's best if you use really juicy, ripe, large strawberries for this recipe.

✳ Berries can be tart as well as sweet, so they are a good new taste for baby to try out. Strawberries can also be great as finger foods, cut up into thin strips or even offered as a large whole strawberry and letting baby go to work on them with their gums (as long as the strawberry will squidge between your finger and thumb – see page 40).

Makes about 1 portion

1. Drain and rinse 40g pre-cooked butter beans. Steam 1 small handful of spinach with the butter beans for about 4 minutes or until the spinach has wilted. Drain and then separate the spinach and butter beans. Blend the spinach for just a few seconds (spinach doesn't mash well).
2. Once cool, use your fingers to slide the insides of the butter beans out of their skins and discard the skin – they are a little tough and large for a young baby to manage.
3. Remove the stalks from 4 medium strawberries (keep 1 large one aside to offer whole as a finger food) and mash them with the butter bean insides with a fork.
4. Add the pureed spinach to the rest of the ingredients and mix well.
5. Serve the spinach, butter bean and strawberry mash alongside some thin slices of strawberry or one large one.

TIP

Don't be afraid to mix and match combinations of flavours that you wouldn't necessarily have together yourself. This stage is all about exploring and giving baby's taste buds a bit of a ride.

If your baby is really enjoying feeding themselves with their hands, steam a few extra butter beans, peel, and – once out of their shells – squash them into balls and let baby dip them into a spinach and strawberry mash.

Red pepper, turkey and spring onion with pasta pieces

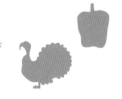

This is more or less the same recipe from Day 20 (see page 96), just with the addition of a few pieces of pasta. This is a great one for helping move baby on to more family-style meals. Pasta is certainly a firm favourite in our house! You can use wholemeal or white versions – fusilli and penne pasta shapes have always been my favourite to offer as early finger food options. If you're worried about baby having whole pieces, try mashing pasta pieces up and mixing them in with the sauce instead.

* Parents are often a little nervous about giving pasta to their baby. However, if you cook it well (not al dente), then it should be super-soft for them to crush between their gums.
* Pasta contains wheat, and so is a potential allergen. Remember to follow the guidelines for introducing allergens on page 56.
* If your little one reacts to the pasta, stop offering it, don't offer it again and book to see your GP.

Makes 1 portion

1. Cook 2–3 pieces of plain, fusilli pasta as per the packet instructions. You could also make pasta for the whole family and take out a few pieces for baby.
2. Cut a red pepper in half and remove the seeds. Brush one half of the pepper lightly with olive oil and pop it under the grill on a high temperature for about 6 minutes or until the skin blackens and starts to crack. Once this happens, remove the pepper from the grill and allow to cool. Remove the skin from the pepper while it's still warm and chop a few slices off and set aside as finger foods.
3. Finely dice the white part of 1 small spring onion and add it to a pan with 50g turkey mince and a little oil, if needed. Cook for about 5 minutes, until the turkey mince is browned all the way through.
4. Chop the rest of the pepper and add to the turkey mince. Blend for a few seconds, allowing for some texture to remain (this one doesn't mash well).
5. Serve the turkey mash with the pasta and the pepper sticks.

TIP

If you find that your baby wants more at this stage, try offering some extra veggie fingers to bulk out the meal a little.

Mushrooms, egg and potato

This recipe is more of a typical breakfast option, but baby can eat it at any time of day. Once you've finished this 30-day guide, you can start focusing on family-friendly breakfasts for baby that work for the whole family, so it's great to introduce that now. There are more breakfast recipes on pages 128–139.

✳ Your baby has hopefully had egg a couple of times now and accepted it, so you can start offering it in more substantial amounts. Yolk and egg white are both fine; there is no need to separate them for baby.

✳ If you want an alternative to egg, try something like black beans or tofu with this dish instead.

Makes about 2 portions

1. Peel about 100g potato and cut into finger-shaped sticks. Steam for 10–12 minutes or until the potato fingers are nice and soft.
2. Meanwhile, boil an egg for 8–10 minutes, making sure it's cooked all the way through. Peel, and cut in half and mash one half. Try to include the rest of the egg in your own meal today, if you can.
3. Peel and roughly slice 40g mushrooms and add to a pan with a little olive oil. Fry for about 5 minutes, until soft and brown. Blend for a few seconds until fairly smooth (mushrooms don't mash well).
4. Put the potato (apart from a few sticks to offer on the side), blended mushroom and mashed egg into a bowl and mash really well with a potato masher. Add a splash of baby's usual milk or some cooking water if you need to loosen it a little.
5. Serve the potato, mushroom and egg mash with the sticks of potato.

MAKING FINGER BALLS
To make this more finger-food-friendly, simply roll all the ingredients into mini balls once cooked. You can bake them in the oven at 200°C for about 20 minutes if you wish, or offer them as they are.

Tomatoes, cannellini beans and basil

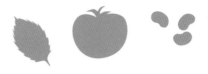

Today is about trying more flavours and what's better than the smell of freshly torn basil? Give your baby a little basil leaf to rub in between their fingers at the start of the meal and encourage them to smell it. Remember offering 'repeated exposures' can mean smelling, touching and feeling the food, and not just eating it (see page 34).

✳ Beans are a great way to offer some protein and iron at mealtimes, but start with small portions and build up gradually to allow baby's digestive system to get used to higher fibre meals.

✳ Tomatoes are such an easy food to offer to baby – I love making bulk tomato sauces and using them for multiple purposes across the week.

✳ You can serve this with some rice, potato or couscous to bulk out the meal if your baby would like more to eat.

Makes about 1 portion

1. Drain and rinse 40g tinned cannellini beans. Add 1 large tomato to a steamer with the beans and cook for 3–4 minutes.
2. Once cooled a little, remove the skin from the tomato (it should peel off very easily). Chop the tomato into slices, discarding any hard bits. Set aside a few slices of tomato to offer as finger foods.
3. Blend the rest of the tomato with 1 fresh basil leaf for just a few seconds (if you blend for too long it'll turn into soup).
4. Mash the beans really well with a fork or a potato masher and then stir them into the tomato and basil mixture.
5. Serve the tomato, bean and basil mash with the tomato slices.

TIP

If your baby is a little windy after eating beans, try offering them in smaller amounts and less often. You can always use protein foods such as nut butters, fish, eggs or meat as replacements.

If you want more finger food options, add some veggie fingers to the meal and use this recipe as a dip, or pour it over some peeled, soft, cooked potatoes. You could also add some mashed potato to the mixture and roll it into mini tomato balls.

Aubergine, chickpeas and plum

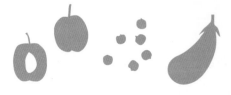

This is a quirky recipe that works well because the neutral or slightly bitter flavour of the aubergine is mixed with the sweeter taste of the plum. It's actually really tasty, so you could spread a little bit on some toast for yourself or add it to porridge.

⁕ Plum is a great option as it's quite tart as well as a little sweet so it adds some complexity to baby's flavour exposures.

⁕ Plums vary a lot in terms of their ripeness. If they are nice and ripe, you might not need to steam them, so you can just chop and add to the mixture.

Makes about 2 portions

1. Cut an aubergine in half lengthways, score the flesh and drizzle over a little olive oil. Pop it in the oven at 200°C for 30–40 minutes, until the flesh is soft and gooey.
2. Peel and destone a plum and slice it into fingers.
3. Rinse and drain 30g tinned chickpeas. Put in a steamer with the plum slices and cook for about 5 minutes, until the plum is nice and soft.
4. Set aside a few of the plum fingers for finger foods.
5. Scoop out the inside of the aubergine and discard the skin. Put the aubergine, plum and chickpeas into a blender and blend for just a few seconds, leaving a little texture.
6. Serve the aubergine, chickpea and plum mash with the plum sticks.

TIP

The skin on plums can be quite tough, so it's good to remove it as it doesn't blend well and it'll be tough for baby to break down without developed chewing skills.

You can add more plum or veggie sticks to this meal for more finger foods.

Banana with oats and peanut butter

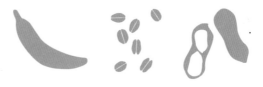

This was always one of my favourite options for Raffy in the early days, especially to take on the go; a small pot of peanut butter with a whole banana and a fork – that's all you need. Adding the oats adds some carbohydrates and extra energy to the dish.

✳ Oats are one of my favourite ingredients for weaning. They are so versatile and you can make them sweet or savoury – check out my other oat recipes on pages 129 and 133–135.

Makes about 1 portion

1. Put 20g oats in a pan with about 100ml water or baby's usual milk.
2. Cook over a low heat for about 5 minutes.
3. Once soft and gooey, add 1 teaspoon of peanut butter and stir well.
4. Serve with a few sticks of banana.

If you find that your baby wants more at this stage, try offering some extra veggie fingers to bulk out the meal a little. Alternatively, mix the oats, ¼ mashed banana and the peanut butter in a bowl and roll into little energy balls. This makes about three balls and is a great way to expose baby to a variety of soft finger foods.

TIP
People always ask about which oats to buy, but any – rolled, ground or flaked – are fine for baby. Just try to get them to the right texture by cooking for a little longer, or grinding them up yourself, if necessary.

Carrot cake porridge

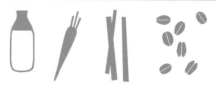

This is one of my most popular recipes to date. I've adapted it here for younger babies and to allow for the introduction of another allergen – cow's milk – which some of you may be trying for the first time. This recipe is a great way to add in a little extra veg in the morning and it tastes pretty good too!

＊ If your baby hasn't had any form of formula milk and you haven't given any dairy products as yet, treat the cow's milk in this recipe as you would with the rest of the allergens and make sure it's the only new food you offer today (leave out the cinnamon, for example) as well as leaving 2–3 days before offering another new allergen.

Makes about 1–2 portions

1. Peel 1 medium carrot (cut a few sticks of the carrot into finger foods if you want to serve some finger foods too). Steam for 12–15 minutes, until soft and mashable.
2. Put 100ml cow's milk and 20g oats in a pan.
3. Once the carrot sticks are cooked, set a few sticks aside, then mash the rest really well with a potato masher. Add them to the pan with the milk and oats and stir well.
4. Cook for about 5 minutes, until the oats thicken and the milk has mostly been absorbed. Add a tiny pinch of cinnamon, if using (see above). Serve in a bowl with a few sticks of cooked carrot.

TIP

It's a good idea to avoid baby getting used to sweet breakfasts all the time. Quite often lots of breakfast options for babies have added sugars or concentrated fruits to make them more appealing. It's absolutely fine to add some fruit in the morning, but try to always think about variety and check out some of the savoury breakfast options in this book (see pages 136–139).

If your baby favours finger foods and self-feeding, pop the Carrot Cake Porridge into mini muffin cases and bake in the oven at 200°C for about 30 minutes to make 2–3 muffins.

Notes

How is your weaning journey one month on?

What are baby's portion sizes like at the end of 30 days?

Are there some foods baby has enjoyed and others
that have been rejected so far?

Write some ideas of new foods you'd like to try.

What allergens will you try next (see page 56)?

_____

_____

_____

_____

_____

_____

_____

_____

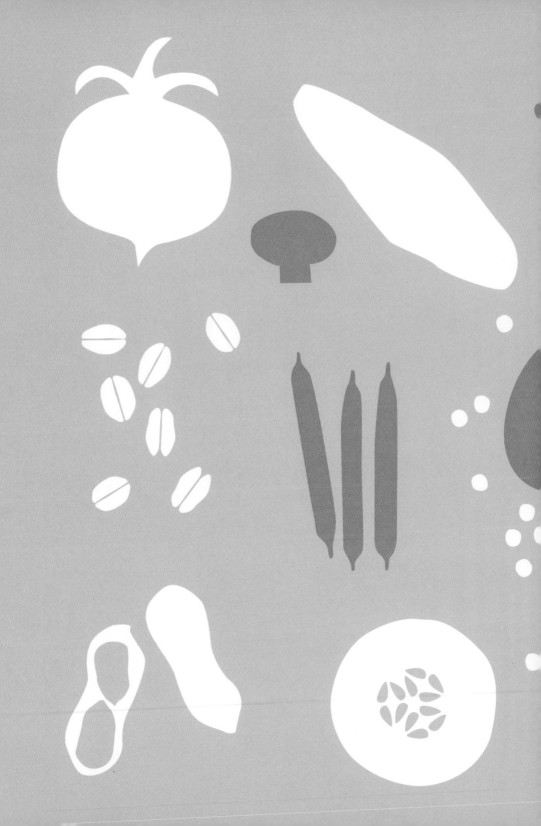

NEXT STEPS OF WEANING

3

Now you've moved through your first 30 days of weaning, I hope you have the confidence to keep exploring a variety and offering your baby plenty of new, exciting dishes. The recipes in Chapter 4 should help you to do just that – they are really focused on family meals and that's what this whole next step in your weaning journey is all about: moving on to family mealtimes. Ultimately, the weaning journey is the process of getting baby from a milk-only diet, to eating a diet that is similar to the rest of the family. So that might mean: exploring textures further (see page 36); baby taking more solids and less milk (see page 118); sharing more of your family cooking with your baby; and thinking about offering baby a 'balanced diet'.

BALANCING BABY'S MEALS

Once your little one is fairly established with their mealtimes and having two or three meals a day, with milk in between, it is a good time to start thinking about how to ensure baby's meals are 'balanced', which means that they contain foods from each of the main food groups:

※ Carbohydrates, such as rice, pasta, potatoes, quinoa and bread.
※ Vegetables and fruits, including frozen and fresh varieties.

✳ Proteins and iron-rich foods, such as beans, lentils, milled nuts, meat, fish and eggs.

✳ Small amounts of full-fat dairy, such as cow's milk, unsweetened yoghurt and cheese, or unsweetened, fortified plant-based alternatives.

Offering foods from each of these main food groups means that, along with any supplements recommended for your baby (see page 65), your little one is likely to be getting everything they need each day to grow and develop well.

Ideally, try to balance the food groups at most meals throughout the day. To help you, I've included a guide on the next page showing how to combine food groups at mealtimes to ensure baby is getting the right variety of foods, nutrients and flavours each day.

For example, why not pair tomatoes + chickpeas + pasta + basil to make a delicious, balanced lunch option.

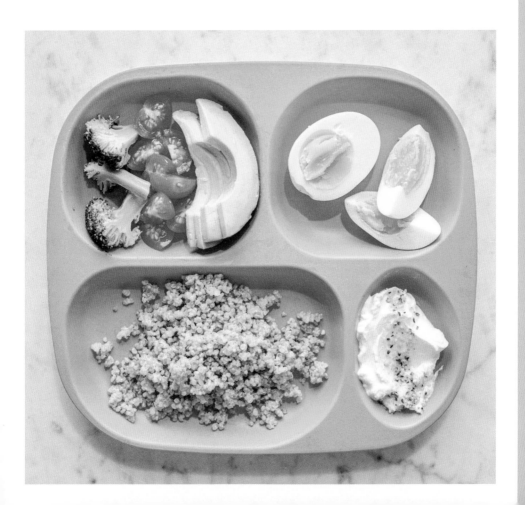

1. LEAD WITH VEGETABLES (& SOME FRUITS)	2. ADD SOME PROTEIN/IRON	3. INCLUDE SOME CARBOHYDRATES	4. ADD EXTRA FLAVOUR
Broccoli	Chicken	Wholegrain pasta	Basil
Courgette	Eggs	White pasta	Oregano
Tomatoes	Beef	Orzo	Thyme
Asparagus	Turkey	Brown rice	Parsley
Carrots	Lamb	White rice	Paprika
Spinach	White fish	Risotto rice	Mixed herbs
Kale	Oily fish	Potatoes	Mixed spices
Cauliflower	Kidney beans	Couscous	Turmeric
Butternut squash	Lentils	Quinoa	Cumin
Aubergine	Chickpeas	Wholemeal bread	Coriander
Sprouts	Hummus	White bread	Cinnamon
Green beans	Butter beans	Buckwheat	Coconut
Sweetcorn	Black beans	Cassava	Garlic
Cabbage	Borlotti beans	Semolina	Onion
Lettuce	Nut butters	Flour	Lemon
Cucumber	Ground nuts	Barley	Lime
Mushroom	Ground seeds	Rye	Cheese
Banana	Tahini	Oats	Black pepper
Berries	Cow's milk	Amaranth	Nutmeg
Orange	Cheese	Polenta	Garam masala
Plums	Tofu	Spelt	Ginger
Peaches	Soya beans		Cardamom
Apples	Peas		
Avocado			

+ HEALTHY FATS

Use oils such as olive oil and rapeseed oil, and unsalted butter/spreads in cooking. You can also offer fats such as cream, yoghurt and nut and seed butters. Healthy fats are also found in avocado.

ALLERGENS

As you move through your weaning journey and on to more complex family meals, remember to continue to offer any new potential allergens one at a time, with a couple of days' gap in between each one. Once they have been accepted and tolerated (with no reaction) continue to offer them regularly, especially the ones you tend to eat as a family. For example, try to offer eggs once a week after they have been accepted and offer around two teaspoons of nut butter each week too.

TEXTURES

Once baby has tackled and mastered purees and mashed foods, it's important to continue to build on baby's eating skills and move through to even more complex textures (see page 39 for more on this). As a general guide, I'd recommend trying to move from minced to chopped textures between around 9 and 12 months of age, so by 12 months, baby is having your family meals, just chopped a little.

PINCER GRIP

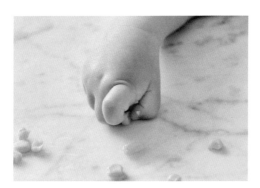

At around nine months of age your baby will start developing their pincer grip (using their forefinger and thumb) to handle smaller pieces of food more easily. Before the pincer grip develops, babies tend to use the palmar grasp and hold objects and foods in their whole hands. It takes a bit of time to develop the pincer grip, and babies need plenty of experience and practice in order to refine this important motor skill. Food is a great way to let them practise this, so you can try chopping up pieces of food such as muffins and pancakes into smaller bits, or offering smaller pieces of soft chicken, soft fruits and foods such as peas for them to experiment with.

MYTH BUST!
—
'My baby should be using utensils well at the age of one'

Don't rush baby to start completely self-feeding with a spoon or expect them to be using cutlery themselves by one year; just give them plenty of opportunities to practise with spoons, cutlery, cups and a variety of finger foods. Role modelling also helps baby to learn some of these self-feeding skills, so be sure to do lots of eating with your baby at their mealtimes.

MILK AMOUNTS

As baby takes larger portions of solids, you might find that their milk intake begins to naturally decline. You can keep offering similar amounts of milk, but try to listen to baby's cues around food and milk so that you let their appetite guide you.

Some babies may need a little help with reducing their milk amounts if you're finding that milk is impacting on baby's food intake at mealtimes. Between 10 and 12 months of age, milk is still an important food for baby, but solid foods begin to make up the majority of nutrients and calories that a baby has, and so it's important that baby doesn't fill up on milk and have little room left for solid foods.

At around 10 months of age, baby only needs around 400ml of formula milk a day, so if your little one is having a lot more than this, it might be worthwhile looking at the mealtime routine to see if you can adjust it slightly. You can absolutely carry on responsively breastfeeding, but just make sure that baby is getting plenty of their calories and nutrients each day from three main meals as well.

The NHS guidance

The NHS guidance on this says: 'At around 7–9 months your baby will gradually move towards eating three meals a day (breakfast, lunch and tea), in addition to their usual milk feeds, which may be around four a day (for example, on waking, after lunch, after tea and before bed).'

At 10 months: 'Your baby should now be having three meals a day (breakfast, lunch and tea), in addition to their usual milk feeds'.

Having a routine around solid foods can really help, as can trying to encourage a nice gap (usually around an hour) between when your baby usually has their milk feed and offering solids. This lets them build up an appetite for food. Ideally, try to offer foods before their milk feeds during the day, so that baby has plenty of appetite for their solid foods.

If you're ever unsure, have a chat with your GP or health visitor about how your baby is doing and get their weight monitored regularly.

TYPICAL MEAL PLAN FOR 7+ MONTHS

Here is a rough guide of what to expect, once three meals are established.

TIME OF DAY	FOOD
Morning	Baby's usual milk breast/bottle
Breakfast	Porridge/cereals/pancakes and veggie/fruit fingers
Nap time	Baby's usual milk breast/bottle before nap
Lunch	Meal with veg, protein and a carbohydrate
Nap time	Baby's usual milk breast/bottle before nap
Dinner	Family-style meals, adapted
Before bed	Baby's usual milk breast/bottle

FOOD REFUSAL

Most of us will go through phases of food refusal with our little ones, whether for a few days, weeks or on and off over the whole journey – it happens. I have had many occasions with Raffy where he went off certain foods and even days and weeks where he ate very little of anything. It's all very normal, so if it happens to you and your little one, try not to worry too much. Think back to my five key principles on page 12 and make sure they are in place (especially the one about staying calm, which I appreciate is hard to master during periods of food refusal!). Try not to get too stressed at mealtimes. Instead, sit with baby, let them play with and explore the food, and get on quietly with eating your own. This takes the pressure off everyone, as well as demonstrating all the ideal behaviours you want to encourage. It's often all that's needed to get your baby or child to show an interest in foods again.

Remember that babies, just like us as adults, will have ups and downs in appetite depending on whether they are growing, ill, teething, tired, distracted, overexcited, over-hungry, reaching milestones, out of their routine etc. They will also have days where they just don't fancy that delicious gourmet meal you've prepared. The only way they can explain that they don't want it is by refusing it.

Keep going!

Don't give up – it can take 10 times for some foods to be accepted. If your little one starts to refuse foods, it's so important not to just take them off the menu – it might just be that they don't feel like broccoli that day, so give it a little rest and try again another day, without comment! They will, of course, ultimately have their own likes and dislikes, just as we do as adults, and that's OK. In the early days, it's important not to limit their likes just yet!

WHAT TO DO WHEN FOOD REFUSAL KICKS IN

○ Continue to do what you normally do, so stick to similar routines and offer similar foods as much as possible.

○ Role model by sitting and eating with your little one as often as you can.

○ Remain calm and avoid drawing lots of undue attention to the food refusal itself.

○ Avoid pressuring baby at mealtimes, including forcing, coaxing or distraction techniques to encourage them to 'eat up'.

○ Listen to their signals as much as you can, and try to respond accordingly (see page 52).

○ Avoid offering alternatives regularly as this can encourage further food refusal.

○ Look at the bigger picture instead of looking day to day or meal to meal. Keep an eye on intakes over a week or so – it's often more reflective of their appetite as a whole.

○ Check the environment at mealtimes – are they calm and relaxed (are you?) when the meal begins? If not, it might be worth trying to change up the mealtime environment.

○ Make sure baby isn't simply too full from milk or grazing on food during the day – this can lead to lower appetites for mealtimes.

○ Be consistent and persistent in your approach with baby. If you respond to food refusal in different ways each time, they won't know what to expect.

○ Look for underlying reasons and, if it's going on a while, check in with your health visitor to see if there could be anything else causing it.

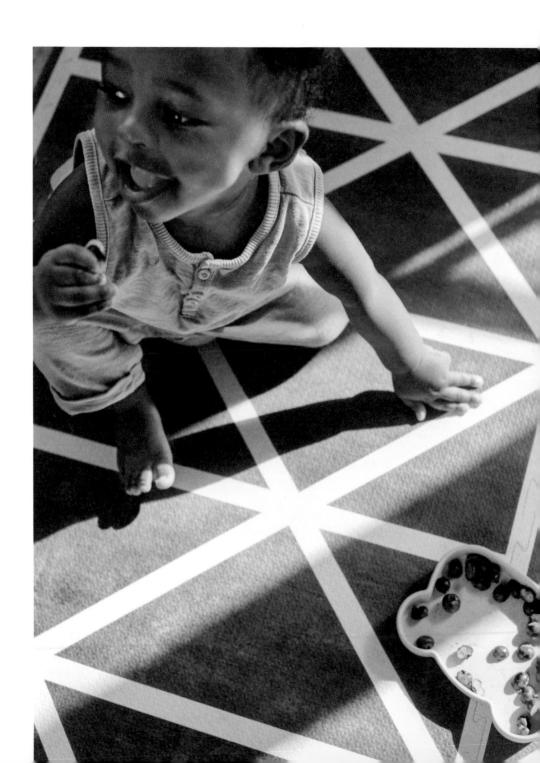

Reaching 12 months

As your baby reaches one year of age, hopefully with the guidance from this book and your own confidence with feeding, your little one will be a seasoned little foodie who has explored a variety of foods and flavours and who can confidently deal with a wide variety of textures. Baby should now be getting most of their calories from their three balanced meals each day, topping up on milk in between these meals and mainly eating the same foods – including all the herbs and spices (but not salt and sugar) – that you eat as a family.

The recipes in the next section will help to give you some ideas for 'what's next'. They may challenge your notion of what it's like to feed a baby, but that's OK. All of the ingredients are safe for babies to have, and you may just need to adapt the textures and portions as your baby develops and moves towards one year of age. The best thing about these recipes is that many of them are for the whole family, so you can continue to have them with your baby/toddler as long as you like and well after your weaning journey has finished. Just remember to season your own portion with salt after you've removed baby's.

I really hope you enjoy them.

'The best thing about
these recipes is that
many of them are
for the whole family'

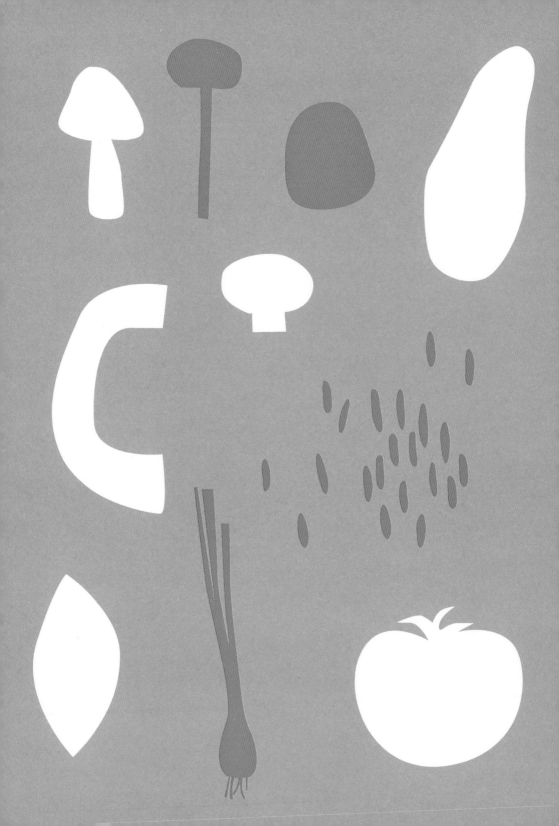

RECIPES

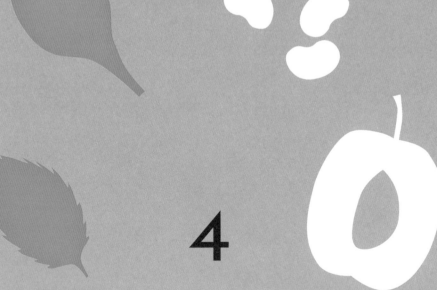

4

I want to keep weaning realistic for parents. I, for one, don't have hours to slave over the hob each day and I know how hard it can be when you have to feed a baby three times a day as well as yourself and the rest of your family. For this reason I've tried to keep these recipes simple and tasty, using ingredients that you're likely to have in your cupboards from one day to the next. The recipes are also easy to put together and adapt, giving you simple meals that can serve your whole family.

Serving sizes will vary, especially as baby moves through their weaning journey and starts eating larger portions, but most leftovers can easily be frozen and you can double many of the recipes to make more when needed.

I've split the recipes into Breakfast, Lunch, Dinner and Finger foods, light bites and puds, rather than specifying ages that they can/should be offered. This is because babies move through weaning at totally different paces; some take to textures and solid pieces of food pretty quickly, while others might be a bit slower. It's all perfectly normal and allowing for flexibility in this book was important to me – no babies follow the exact same path (see page 22 for more on this).

Some of the recipes are just for baby, some are for baby and a parent, and some are for a larger family. In those cases, just a little extra chopping, mashing or mincing might be all that's needed to make them suitable for your baby. It's important to follow your baby's lead and offer them food textures and sizes that you and they are comfortable with, rather than following particular 'stages' that might not suit your baby's own journey.

ADAPTING THE RECIPES TO SUIT YOU

If you're raising your baby as a vegetarian, pescatarian or a vegan, you will find plenty of recipes here that will work for you. I also explain how to adapt the meat-based recipes, and you can swap in beans and pulses wherever you like. From six months, you can use unsweetened plant milks in baby's food (see page 26). If you're choosing plant-based options for milk, cheese and yoghurt, choose those fortified with nutrients where possible and opt for unsweetened versions. Try plant-based spreads and oils instead of butter, coconut milk instead of yoghurt and nutritional yeast for a cheesy flavour.

EGG ALTERNATIVES

If a recipe calls for eggs, you can swap in one of these alternatives, if you prefer. Each of these options is the equivalent of one egg:

* **1 ripe banana, mashed.** This is great in recipes such as pancakes.
* **1 tablespoon ground flaxseeds or chia seeds**, with 3 tablespoons of water. Mix together and set aside for 15 minutes. This works well in baking, such as muffins.
* **Plant-based egg replacers**: You can buy egg replacer products from health food shops (choose one without added salt), and they work well in baking.
* **Aquafaba**: This is the liquid from a tin of chickpeas; 3 tablespoons is about 1 egg. Whip it until it forms stiff peaks, and use for meringues and bakes.

breakfast

Breakfast has *always* been Raffy's favourite meal of the day. Young babies often wake up from their sleep super-hungry and once they stop having milk in the morning (around 10–12 months), their hunger can turn to 'hanger' as they are waiting for that first meal. This happened with Raffy, but his appetite in the morning has definitely calmed now he is a little older.

Having some quick go-to brekkie options, such as porridge, fortified cereals and toast and toppings, can be an easy win. The pancakes on pages 129 and 138 are also fab as you can freeze them and defrost in the fridge the night before so you've got a quick breakfast when you need it. Pina Colada Overnight Oats (see page 135) is made the night before in about five minutes so it's ready to serve to those hangry monsters first thing!

BLUEBERRY OATY PANCAKES

Prep: 2 minutes
Cook: 10 minutes
Makes: 10–12 mini pancakes

I love a pancake recipe and here I wanted to come up with a really quick, fuss-free option that you can make in a rush and even eat on the go or while out and about. Try making these into tiny bite-sized pancakes, which are perfect for young babies to practise their self-feeding skills.

150g oats
1 free-range egg
1 tsp baking powder
1–2 tbsp chopped nuts
   (any nuts are fine)
150ml milk of choice
100g blueberries
a drizzle of oil, for cooking

1. Put all the ingredients (except the oil) into a blender and blend until smooth.
2. Heat the oil in a frying pan and, once hot, add a thick dollop of your pancake mixture into the middle of the pan. You will be cooking 8–10 so if you have space, add a few more pancakes to the pan.
3. Once it's browning nicely, flip your pancake and cook it on the other side. Repeat until you have used all the batter. Cut a pancake into strips for baby.
4. Serve with a yoghurt dip and some fruity fingers or my Berry Pancake Topping recipe on page 139.

NUTTY FRENCH TOAST

When it comes to feeding babies and children, I'm always trying to find ways to add extra nutrients into meals and recipes. This recipe does just that – a French toast recipe with a nutty twist, and it really doesn't take long to make either!

Prep: 5 minutes
Cook: 10 minutes
Serves: 2 (double the ingredients if making for you too)

a drizzle of olive oil
1 free-range egg
a pinch of cinnamon
1–2 tsp 100 per cent
    peanut butter, smooth
1 slice bread
plain yoghurt and berry pancake
    topping (see page 139) or mashed
    berries, to serve (optional)

1. Heat the oil in a pan over a medium heat.
2. Whisk the egg in a bowl with the cinnamon.
3. Spread the peanut butter on one side of the bread and then dip both sides of the bread in the egg mixture. Leave for a good few seconds on each side to soak up some of the egg.
4. Add your bread to the pan and cook on either side for about 3 minutes, until slightly browning and the egg is cooked.
5. Cut the toast into strips for baby to feed themselves. If you like, serve with a dollop of yoghurt and berry pancake topping as a dip.

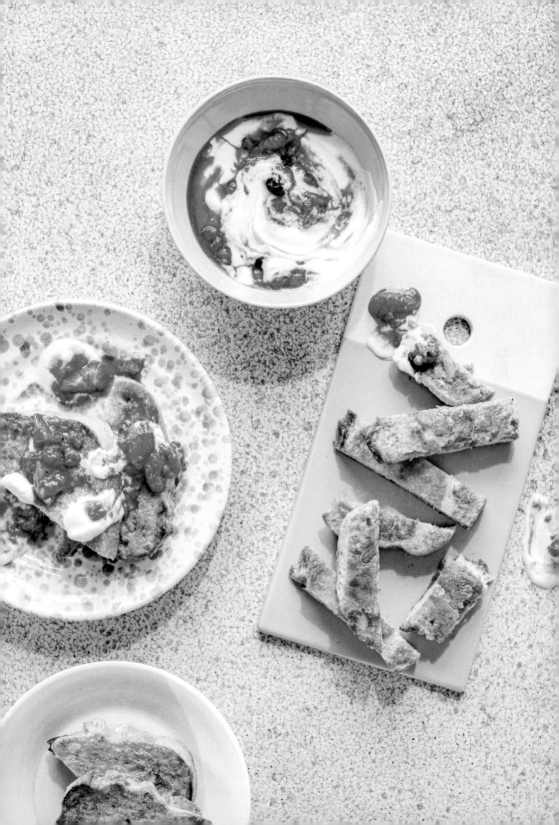

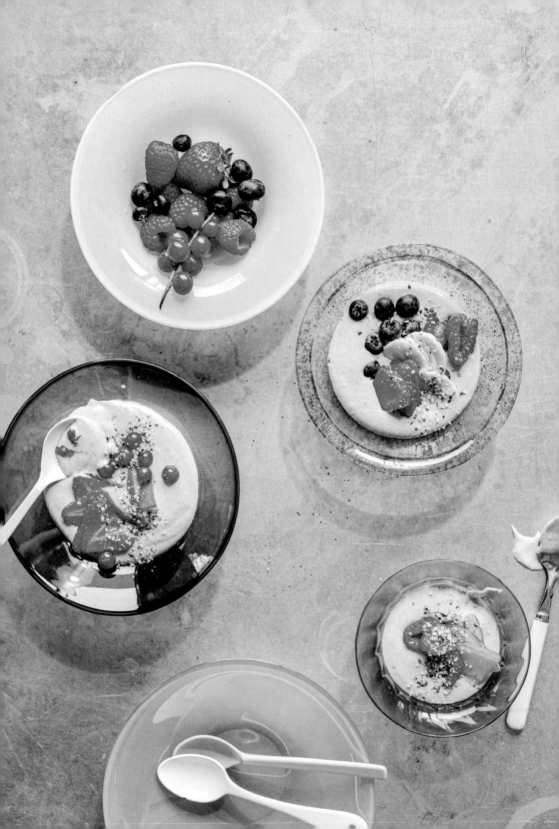

BABY'S FIRST SMOOTHIE BOWL

This breakfast is super-quick to whizz together and is perfect served with milled seeds and fresh fruit fingers on top for baby to practise some of those self-feeding and dipping skills. It's a nutrient-packed breakfast for you too.

Prep: 2 minutes
Serves: 1 baby, 1 adult

1 medium banana
2 tsp 100 per cent peanut butter, smooth
2 heaped tbsp Greek yoghurt
25g oats
fresh fruits, sliced (strawberry
    is lovely) and 1 tsp milled seeds,
    to serve (optional)

1. Pop everything into a blender (except the fruit and seeds to serve, if using) and blend for a few seconds until it's well mixed. If it needs thickening up, add a few more oats.
2. Serve in a bowl with some milled seeds sprinkled on top and some sliced fruits of your choice.

THE ULTIMATE CARROT CAKE PORRIDGE

Prep: 5 minutes
Cook: 10 minutes
Serves: 2

OK, so Carrot Cake Porridge features in this book already, and it's also one of my most popular recipes to date, but this is the ultimate version just for this book. I like to think it's a bit of a classic of mine, and something that I hope parents will offer to their babies for years.

Carrot Cake Porridge is a fab way to get some veggies in in the morning and allows us, as parents, to vary from the 'sweet' that is so often associated with breakfast time.

20g carrot (about ¼ carrot), peeled and finely grated
40g porridge oats
150ml milk of choice
a pinch of cinnamon
a tiny pinch of nutmeg
1 tsp nut butter (optional)
2 tsp cream cheese, to serve
zest of 1 orange, to serve
a few slices of pear, cut into fingers, to serve (optional)

✳ For younger babies you can grind the oats before cooking and puree the cooked carrot, if you prefer. For most babies cooked whole oats are fine and offer a nice texture for them to try.

1. Put the grated carrot into a pan. Cook for 2–3 minutes over a medium heat, just to slightly warm and soften the carrot.
2. Add the oats, milk, cinnamon, nutmeg and nut butter (if using), and cook over a low heat for about 5 minutes, until the porridge starts to thicken.
3. Once ready, transfer to your breakfast bowls and top each with 1 teaspoon of cream cheese and a sprinkle of orange zest – stir it through to make the final porridge nice and creamy.
4. Serve with a couple of sticks of pear fingers if you like.

✳ **Leftover porridge muffins**
Any untouched leftover porridge can be put in muffin cases and baked in the oven for 30 minutes at 200°C to make muffins.

PINA COLADA OVERNIGHT OATS

Prep: 2 minutes (the night before)
Serves: 1 baby, 1 adult

I'm super-proud of this recipe, mainly because it's so delicious and refreshing – the pineapple is a real taste of the Caribbean! Overnight oats are also fab when you need a quick morning option, so don't be afraid to use this recipe as a base for lots of other toppings too! I use fresh pineapple, but you can also use tinned in juice.

75g oats
75g pineapple, chopped or blended (depending on baby's stage), plus extra to decorate
1½ tsp desiccated coconut, plus extra to decorate
1 tsp chia seeds
About 100ml milk of choice

1. Mix the oats, pineapple, coconut and chia seeds in a bowl and stir together well. Pour over just enough milk (about 100ml) to cover and pop in the fridge.
2. In the morning stir in a little more milk if needed and top with a sprinkle of coconut and a few soft pieces of pineapple as finger food.

✳ If you want to make this just for baby, use about 30g oats and 30g pineapple for a baby-sized breakfast.

CHEESY QUINOA PORRIDGE

Prep: 5 minutes
Cook: 15 minutes
Serves: 1 baby, 1 adult

Don't be put off by the title – this recipe is delicious! I love the idea of varying things up at breakfast, and if you're stuck in a porridge rut, offering something like this can work wonders! This recipe takes a little more time, but you could try using quinoa flakes instead of dry quinoa for the porridge, which speeds things up a lot.

100g quinoa, rinsed and drained
200ml milk of choice
20g Cheddar cheese, grated
1 free-range egg, to serve (optional)
a drizzle of oil, for cooking
100g mushrooms, sliced
200g cherry tomatoes, sliced
50g spinach

✳ You can blend the veggies together for younger babies who aren't able to cope with these textures yet, and serve it mixed in with the cheesy quinoa.

1. Put the quinoa into a pan with the milk and bring to the boil. Once boiling, reduce the heat to low, cover with a lid and cook for 10–15 minutes, until the quinoa is cooked and fluffy (add a little extra milk if needed). Stir through the Cheddar cheese.
2. Meanwhile, if you are having an egg, boil the egg for about 8 minutes, until cooked.
3. Meanwhile, heat the oil in a large pan, add the mushrooms and cook for about 5 minutes. Add the tomatoes to one side of the pan and cook everything for a further 5 minutes. Once the mushrooms are browned and starting to crisp, add the spinach, stir everything gently and cook for 2 minutes, until the spinach is wilted.
4. Chop up some of the mushrooms, tomatoes and spinach for baby.
5. Put the cheesy quinoa in your breakfast bowls with the mushroom, tomato and spinach mixture on top.
6. Cut the egg in half, if using, and serve one half chopped for baby and one half whole for you.

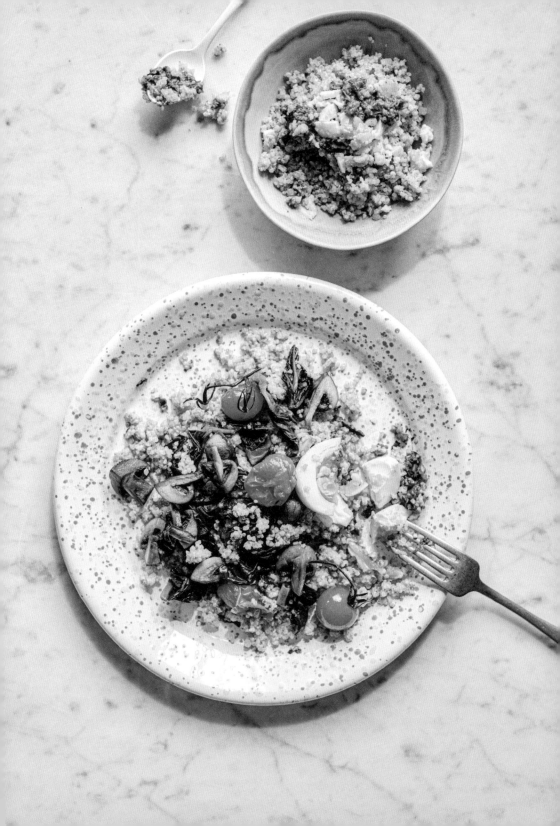

BABY PANCAKES – SWEET AND SAVOURY!

Prep: 5 minutes
Cook: 10 minutes
Serves: 8 –10 pancakes

I love pancakes, but I don't think they always need to be covered in maple syrup (not ideal for babies) and super-sweet. So here I've taken a basic, quick and easy American-style pancake recipe that's perfect for babies as it has no added sugar or salt, and then created some sweet and savoury topping ideas so you can vary how you offer them to baby. Pancakes don't just have to be for brekkie either – they are a great meal to take on the go and they freeze well so you can make them in bulk and get them out for those rushed mornings.

BASIC PANCAKE RECIPE:

250g self-raising flour
1 tsp baking powder
1 free-range egg
300ml milk of choice
a little drizzle of oil, for cooking

✳ If baby doesn't eat eggs, try some of the egg replacement options on page 127.

1. Sift the flour into a large bowl with the baking powder and make a well in the middle.
2. Crack the egg into a jug, add the milk and whisk it together.
3. Add the milk mixture to the well in your flour and whisk together until you have a smooth batter.
4. Heat the oil in a frying pan and, once hot, add a thick dollop of your pancake mixture into the middle of the pan.
5. Once it's browning nicely, flip your pancake and cook it on the other side. Repeat until you have used all the batter. Cut a pancake into strips for baby to grab as finger food.

✳ **Note:**
I use rapeseed oil or olive oil for cooking. Use whichever you like!

BERRY PANCAKE TOPPING

Prep: 2 minutes
Cook: 5 minutes
Serves: 2

Berries can be very tart but it's great to expose your baby to different flavours so don't feel you need to sweeten this to remove the tartness. Including some yoghurt will help to tone it down a little, but actually some babies love the taste of a berry coulis just like this – Raffy still loves it to this day! Frozen berries are so convenient and great value too; we always have a bag in the freezer.

100g frozen or fresh forest
    fruits/berries
natural yoghurt, to serve
a few sprigs of mint, to decorate

1. Heat the berries in a pan over a medium heat for about 5 minutes, until they start to bubble a little and turn mushy.
2. Mash a little with a fork and leave to cool.
3. Serve on top of the pancakes with a dollop of yoghurt and a sprig of mint, if you like, to decorate your adult portion.

✳ You can also chop fresh mint finely and add it to the berry mix for a different flavour.

EGG AND SPINACH PANCAKE TOPPING

Prep: 5 minutes
Cook: 10 minutes
Serves: 3, or 1 adult, 1 baby

There is no reason why pancakes have to be sweet and topping them with some veggies is a perfect way to get baby eating veg in the morning too.

---

1 tsp olive oil
10g leek or spring onion
    (white part only), finely chopped
1 medium ripe tomato, finely chopped
10g spinach, finely chopped
3 free-range eggs
a large pinch of oregano
black pepper (optional)

1. Heat the oil in a pan over a high heat and add the leek or spring onion. Cook for about 5 minutes, until softened, then add the tomato and cook for 2 minutes before adding the spinach.
2. In a bowl, whisk the eggs together with the oregano and a small grind of black pepper (if using) and then pour into the vegetable mix.
3. Stir everything together to scramble the eggs, and cook for about 3 minutes, until they are fully cooked. Serve piled on top of your pancakes.

✳ You can offer the scrambled egg mixture on a spoon or as finger food for baby to pick up.

lunch

When I'm at home, lunch often has to be a quick and easy option. I often fall back on simply looking at what's in the fridge and making Raffy finger food plates of whatever is available. I did this from when he was a really young age as I found cooking three meals was a little too much every day!

However, if you're feeling more experimental I've put together some of my favourite lunch options here. Some take a little longer to prepare for those days when baby has a nice long nap, and others are simple and quick options that you can throw together in minutes. Most are also perfect for the whole family, so you can double or halve the ingredients in these recipes, as needed.

TOFU FRIED RICE

Prep: 2 minutes
Cook: 30 minutes
Serves: 2 babies, 1 adult

This dish makes a lovely lunch, or is the perfect addition to a curry! If you use ready-cooked rice, it's also super-quick and easy to make. A great one for a fast lunch option. Remember that sesame is an allergen so follow the allergen guidelines on page 56.

75g brown rice
1 tsp sesame oil
2 spring onions, well chopped
100g tofu (or 2 free-range eggs, whisked)
1 tsp ground ginger
1 tsp garlic paste
100g frozen veggies e.g. peas, carrots and broccoli

✳ You can always mash the ingredients together well with the back or a fork, or blend with a little extra cooking water or milk, if needed.

1. Cook the rice as per the packet instructions (about 30 minutes).
2. Heat the sesame oil in a large frying pan over a medium heat.
3. Add the spring onions and cook for 3–4 minutes. Crumble in the tofu (or whisked eggs) followed by the ginger, garlic and frozen vegetables.
4. Stir well and cook for about 5 minutes, until the vegetables are defrosted and well mixed.
5. Lastly, drain the rice and add it to the pan, stirring well for a further 2 minutes.

✳ Serve with a little yoghurt or some hummus on the side. For adults, this works well with a few drops of soy sauce.

QUICK QUESADILLAS

Prep: 5 minutes
Cook: 15 minutes
Serves: 1 baby, 1 adult

I love making these 'wrap pizzas' – they are often a go-to option when I've run out of ideas, want something tasty, filling and also veg-packed. As with many of the recipes throughout this book, the veggies used here are just ideas – you can use whatever you have in your fridge.

2 tsp olive oil
40g (about ¼) leek, well chopped
60g (about ¼) aubergine, well chopped
1 large beef tomato, well chopped
100g tinned butter beans,
    roughly chopped
½ tsp ground coriander
½ tsp paprika
1 tbsp tomato puree
2 large or 4 mini wraps
40g Cheddar cheese, grated

✳ If you have a younger baby who may struggle with the lumpy veg, you can always blend the veggie ingredients together before spreading on the wraps. Younger babies might not be able to hold the wraps and eat them as we do as adults, but these offer a great way to practise those self-feeding skills.

1. Heat the oil in a pan over a medium heat and, once hot, add the leek and cook for about 5 minutes. Add the aubergine and tomato and cook for a further 5 minutes, until softened. Add the butter beans, coriander and paprika, and stir it all through nicely. Cook for another 2 minutes or so.
2. Put the tomato puree in a small bowl and add 2 tablespoons of water to make a more liquidy paste.
3. Put a large wrap in a frying pan and evenly spread some of the tomato puree mixture over, like a pizza.
4. Add a large spoonful of the veggie mix to half of the wrap and top with a little grated cheese. Fold the wrap and squash it down really well. Pop it under a hot grill for a few minutes to brown the top and melt the cheese. If using mini wraps, pop 1 in the pan, put the tomato puree, veggies and cheese in the middle and put another wrap on top. Repeat with the remaining wraps and ingredients.

✳ This also works really well with shredded chicken mixed in with the veggies.

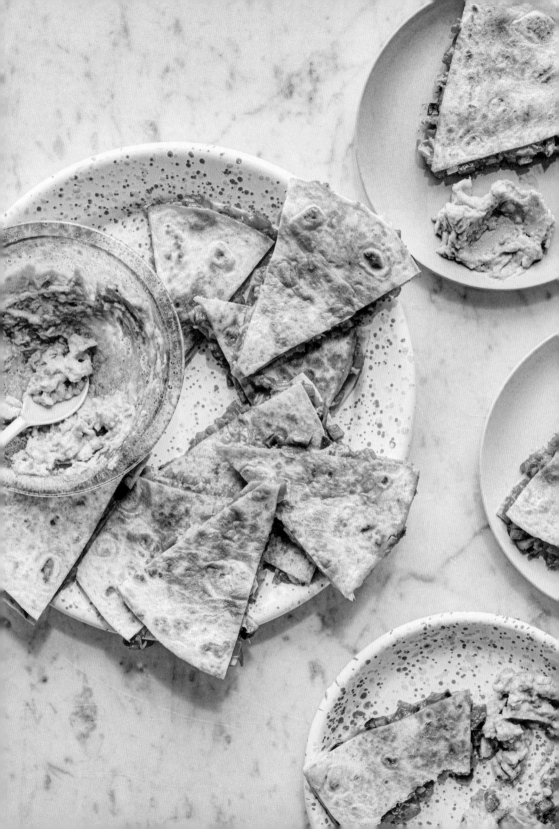

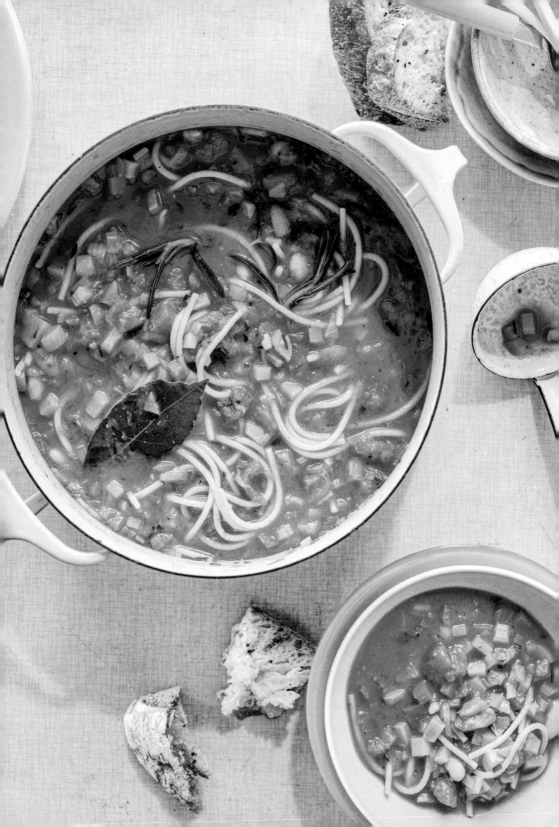

MISTER STRONE SOUP

Prep: 10 minutes
Cook: 40 minutes
Serves: a family of 4

This is a meal that I grew up on. My mum is a seasoned pro at minestrone and, although initially Raffy wasn't the biggest fan of soup, once Grandma made him her minestrone he couldn't get enough, and he still loves it to this day. He calls it 'Mister Strone'! Hope your family enjoy this just as much as we do – it's a really wholesome, family meal.

1 tbsp olive oil
1 small onion, diced
1 garlic clove, finely chopped
2 sticks celery, well chopped
2 carrots, well chopped
1 tbsp tomato puree
1 bay leaf
2 tsp mixed herbs
2 sprigs of fresh rosemary, chopped,
    or 1 tsp dried rosemary
1 small red pepper, deseeded and
    well chopped
1 x 400g tin chopped tomatoes
800ml water or vegetable stock
    (see page 197)
60g spaghetti
200g tinned cannellini beans (chop
    a little for younger babies)

1. Heat the olive oil in a large pan, add the onion and cook for 5 minutes.
2. Add the garlic, celery and carrots and cook for a further 5 minutes, until they start to soften.
3. Add the tomato puree, bay leaf, mixed herbs, rosemary, red pepper and tomatoes, then pour in the water or stock.
4. Stir and then bring to a simmer and cook for 15 minutes with the lid on. For young babies, you can blend some of the mixture after this stage if you like.
5. Snap the spaghetti into pieces and add to the pan with the beans. Simmer for about 15 minutes, until the pasta is cooked. Remove the bay leaf and the fresh rosemary (if used) before serving with some nice warm bread.

✳ You can always blend or mash this minestrone soup for younger babies, but most of the veggies in this are super-soft and it's a good way of starting to expose baby to more textures, lumps and chunks in their foods as they move towards a year old.

EASY HUMMUS PINWHEELS

Prep: 5 minutes
Makes: 12 mini pinwheels

I love making these no-cook pinwheels, using just a tortilla wrap. You can vary the ingredients in these wraps, so they are a great option for a fridge raid. Tuna and salmon mashed up work well in a wrap too. You can always swap the tortilla wrap for my Chickpea Flatbread recipe on page 193.

1 tortilla wrap
1 tbsp Chickpea Dip (see page 193)
½ small avocado, destoned, skin removed and mashed
a few spinach leaves
a little grated cheese (optional)

1. Spread the wrap with the Chickpea Dip and lay the avocado and spinach leaves on top. Sprinkle the cheese on top, if using.
2. Roll the wrap together tightly and cut the wrap widthways with a sharp knife into little wheels. Serve to baby as a perfect finger food meal along with some veggie sticks.

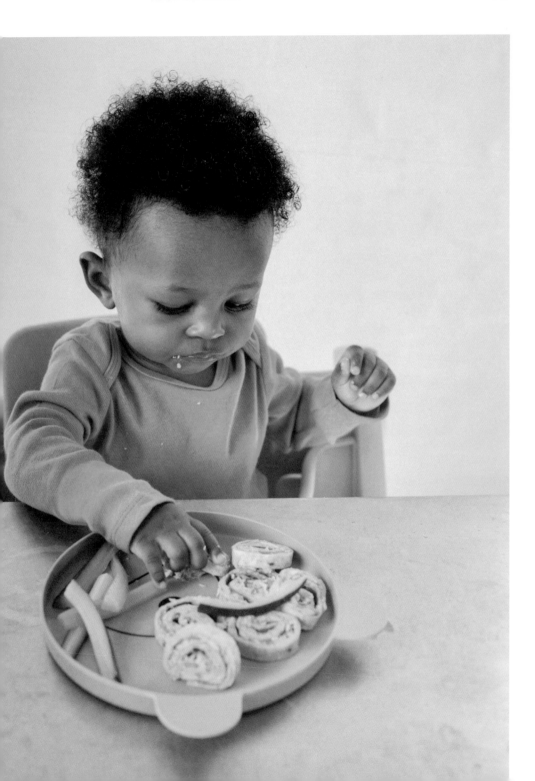

TUNA OPEN SANDWICH

Prep: 2 minutes
Cook: 2 minutes
Serves: 1

This is a very quick and perfectly balanced meal for baby, including carbohydrates, veggies, dairy and proteins. I love making these when I'm in a rush as they're so quick and easy and are a great alternative to tuna mayo. You can always use dairy-free yoghurt if your little one doesn't eat dairy.

1 English muffin
80g tinned tuna (in spring water), drained
2 tbsp natural yoghurt
2 tbsp tinned sweetcorn, drained
2 sticks of cucumber, with skin removed

1. Slice the English muffin in half and pop it in the toaster to lightly toast. Use the other half another day or for yourself!
2. Mix the tuna, yoghurt and sweetcorn together in a bowl and then spread the mixture over one half of the toasted muffin. Cut the muffin half into finger shapes so it is easier for baby to manage.
3. Serve with the sticks of cucumber.

SUPER GREEN FRITTATA

Prep: 5 minutes
Cook: 25 minutes
Serves: 2 babies, 1 adult

Frittatas are such a perfect lunch option as they can be super-quick and simple to bash together. This recipe is easy, but it has a few added ingredients to really make it taste good and to get some extra veggies in for baby and you! I have used asparagus here, but if it's not in season, broccoli is lovely too.

100g potatoes, peeled and
   roughly chopped
100g asparagus, chopped into
   2cm pieces, woody stems removed
2 tsp olive oil
½ onion, roughly chopped
3–4 free-range eggs
a small handful of spinach, well chopped
50g frozen peas
3 mint leaves, roughly chopped
40g Cheddar cheese, grated
black pepper (optional)

✳ If you are making this just for baby, you will only need about one-quarter of the ingredients, but it is lovely for your lunch too. It keeps well in the fridge for the next day too.
✳ Simply mash the mixture together well for younger babies or serve sticks of frittata as finger foods.

1. Put the potatoes in a pan with water, bring to a simmer and cook for 10–12 minutes, until softened. Add the asparagus to the potato water for the last 5 minutes of cooking. Drain, separate the asparagus and set both aside.
2. Meanwhile, heat the oil in a frying pan and, once warm, add the onion and cook for about 5 minutes, until softened.
3. Add the potatoes and cook for another 5 minutes. Meanwhile, heat the grill to its highest setting.
4. While this is cooking, crack the eggs into a bowl, and whisk them really well with a few grinds of black pepper (if using).
5. Add the spinach, peas and cooked asparagus to the pan.
6. Pour the eggs into the pan and make sure they cover the base of the pan and most of the veggies. Add the mint leaves to the mixture. Cook the frittata for a few minutes, until firm at the edges, and then sprinkle the cheese on top.
7. Pop the frittata under the grill for 5 minutes, until the egg is cooked all the way through and the cheese is bubbling away.

SWEET POTATO AND GINGER FISHCAKES

Prep: 15 minutes
Cook: 35 minutes
Makes: about 8 mini fishcakes

Fishcakes have always been one of Raffy's favourites and I've created multiple fishcake recipes over time. This one is brand new and I love the combination of sweet potato and ginger – they go so well together. Don't be afraid to add a little more ginger or lime if you like and make sure not to add any liquid from the fish to the mash.

200g white fish (such as cod, coley or haddock)
1 thumb-sized piece of fresh root ginger, finely chopped
1 garlic clove, peeled and finely chopped
1 lime, zested and cut in half
400g sweet potato, peeled and roughly chopped into chunks
20g fresh coriander, finely chopped
2 spring onions, finely chopped
2 tbsp plain flour
100g breadcrumbs (about 2 slices bread, blended into breadcrumbs)
1 free-range egg
a drizzle of oil, for frying

＊ You can always mash the fishcakes for younger babies or offer as fish sticks for BLW.

1. Preheat the oven to 200°C. Place a large sheet of tin foil on to a baking tray.
2. Add the fish to the middle of the foil, sprinkle over the ginger, garlic, lime zest and the juice of half the lime.
3. Wrap the foil up around the fish to create a parcel, then put the tray in the oven for 10–15 minutes or until the fish is cooked through. Once cooked, open the parcel and leave to cool.
4. Meanwhile, boil the sweet potato for about 10 minutes, until soft. Drain and leave to dry in a sieve for a few minutes, then mash.
5. Once the fish is cool to touch, flake it into the mashed sweet potato. Add the coriander and spring onions and, using your hands, gently squeeze the fish and potato together to combine.
6. Sprinkle the flour over a plate and place the breadcrumbs on another plate. Whisk the egg in a shallow bowl.
7. Shape the fish mixture into 8 fishcakes then, one at a time, coat them in the flour, then dip in the egg. Then dip them in the breadcrumbs, patting the crumbs in so that they stick.
8. Put the fishcakes in the oven and bake for about 20 minutes.

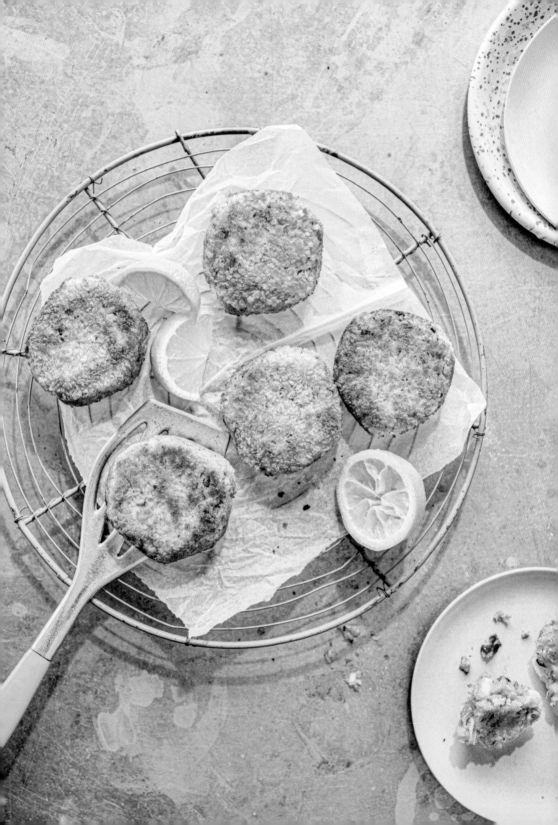

MAC AND CHEESE WITH KALE AND CAULIFLOWER

Who doesn't love mac and cheese? This recipe is delicious – I'm a big fan and it's a great way of getting some cheesy flavours into baby's diet. There are plenty of textures in this to get baby experimenting and practising their self-feeding skills. Don't be afraid to vary the veggies that you use; mushrooms, sweetcorn and spinach all work perfectly in this dish too.

Prep: 5 minutes
Cook: 30 minutes
Serves: 2 babies, 1 adult

150g macaroni pasta
(or wholegrain fusilli)
a large handful of kale, finely
chopped (stems removed)
100g cauliflower (about ¼ of a head),
chopped into small manageable
pieces for baby
20g unsalted butter
20g plain flour
285ml milk of choice (full-fat cow's
milk or fortified, unsweetened oat
milk work well)
¼ tsp garlic granules
¼ tsp nutritional yeast (optional)
60g Cheddar cheese, grated

* All the ingredients should be nice and soft and manageable for a baby who has moved through textures well, but you can always mash or blend, if needed. Add a little extra milk to loosen if blending. Offer with a few solid pieces of pasta and cauliflower as finger foods on the side.

1. Cook the pasta in boiling water for about 5 minutes, then add the kale and cauliflower and cook for a further 5 minutes, until the pasta is cooked and the veggies soft. Drain and leave to one side.
2. Preheat the oven to 200°C, or the grill to high.
3. Put the butter into a large pan and allow to melt over a medium heat.
4. Add the flour and stir well to make a 'roux' (a kind of paste).
5. Gradually add the milk, stirring all the while as it gradually thickens. This can take a little time, so be patient.
6. Once thick, take off the heat and add the garlic granules, nutritional yeast (if using) and 40g of the cheese. Stir well until the cheese has melted.
7. Add the pasta, kale and cauliflower to the cheese sauce and stir well. Transfer to an ovenproof dish and then sprinkle over the rest of the cheese.
8. Cook in the oven or grill for 10–15 minutes, until the cheese has browned on top.

ROAST VEG AND GIANT COUSCOUS

Prep: 10 minutes
Cook: 25 minutes
Serves: a family of 4

Giant couscous is great for babies, helping them to explore new textures, and it always tastes delicious. This is a perfect recipe for the whole family and works well with some cream cheese or pasteurised hard cheese crumbled on top. Cut the vegetables into sticks or chop, depending on what stage your baby is at.

1 courgette, cut into sticks
 or well chopped
1 red pepper, deseeded and
 cut into sticks or well chopped
1 yellow pepper, deseeded and
 cut into sticks or well chopped
200g cherry tomatoes, quartered
a drizzle of olive oil, for cooking
150g giant couscous

For the dressing
2 tbsp olive oil
1 tsp cumin
1 heaped tsp tomato puree
juice of ½ lime
a small grind of black pepper

1. Preheat the oven to 200°C.
2. Put the chopped vegetables into a baking tray, drizzle with the olive oil and roast in the oven for 20–25 minutes or until everything is cooked and golden.
3. Meanwhile, cook the giant couscous according to the packet instructions (about 8 minutes); drain, then set aside.
4. Whisk together all of the dressing ingredients.
5. Put the roasted vegetables, giant couscous and dressing in a large bowl and mix it all together.

✳ Adults can add a little cayenne pepper to the dressing for a spicier kick!

✳ If baby is younger you can offer the veggies as finger food sticks, but for an older baby experimenting more with minced and chopped textures, you can chop the veggies up into smaller pieces to add texture into their food.
✳ You can mash or blend the veggies with the sauce for younger babies if you prefer, and serve alongside the soft giant couscous.

GREEK MEZE

Prep: 15 minutes
Cook: 25 minutes
Serves: a family of 4

I adore Greek food and this Greek-style meze dish is perfect as a finger food-style buffet for the whole family. This recipe uses a few recipes from other parts of the book, so you may have to do some jumping around, but it's well worth it as everything goes together so well.

100g pasteurised feta cheese
1 courgette, cut into batons or slices
1 red pepper, cut into batons or slices
3–4 pitta breads
1 beef tomato, sliced
a drizzle of olive oil
Falafel (see page 167), to serve
Aubergine Dip (see page 193), to serve

✳ Serve to baby as a little finger food buffet but only offer a tiny taste of feta as it's super-salty!

1. Preheat the grill to high and the oven to 200°C.
2. Wrap the feta cheese in tin foil, place it on a baking tray and bake in the oven for 20 minutes. Remove it from the tin foil and grill for a further 5 minutes (this gives it a nice crispy topping).
3. Meanwhile, grill the courgette and red pepper for about 10 minutes, turning halfway through. Once the peppers and courgettes are cooked, cool and remove the skin if needed for younger babies.
4. Toast the pittas lightly and then chop into triangles.
5. Drizzle a little olive oil over the sliced tomato and set aside.
6. Serve all the ingredients on different plates in the middle of the table.

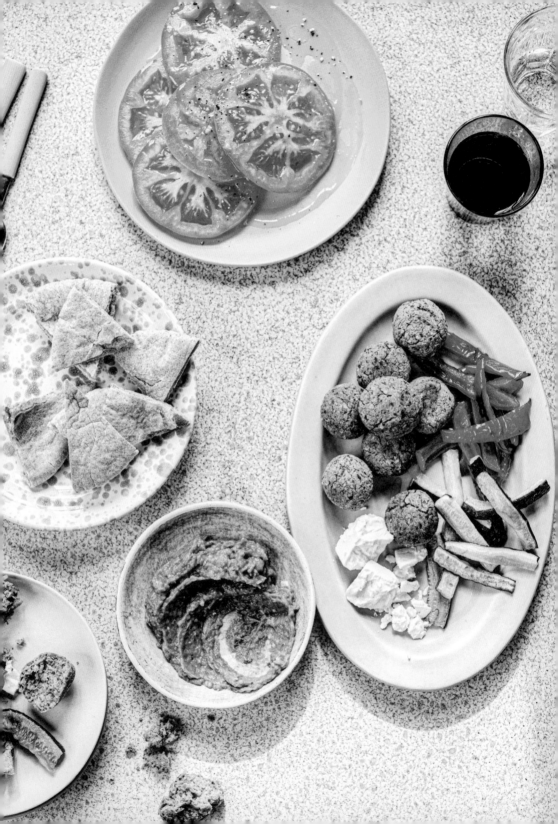

SALMON PESTO PASTA

Pesto pasta is such a quick and easy meal for babies. It's a great way of exposing them to nuts as well as a variety of flavours too. This recipe adds a little extra in too with the grilled salmon!

Prep: 2 minutes
Cook: 20 minutes
Serves: 2

For the pesto (makes enough
   for about 10 servings)
50g basil
50g spinach
20g nuts (cashews, walnuts
   or pine nuts work well)
20g Cheddar cheese, grated
juice of ½ lemon
50ml olive oil

For the salmon pasta
40g dried fusilli pasta
2–3 spears of asparagus, woody stems
   removed, cut or whole (optional)
a drizzle of olive oil, for cooking
½ salmon fillet (skinless and boneless)

✳ For young babies you can mash the pasta and salmon really well or simply offer some pasta, salmon and asparagus fingers with the pesto dip. If you want to blend this a little, you may need a small splash of water to help loosen the ingredients.
✳ Don't offer both salmon and nuts together if it's the first time that baby is trying either foods.

1. Put all the pesto ingredients in a food processor or blender and blitz until smooth. Set to one side.
2. Cook the pasta according to the packet instructions, about 10 minutes. If using, add the asparagus spears to the pan for the last 5 minutes.
3. Meanwhile, heat the olive oil in a non-stick frying pan over a medium heat. Once hot, add the salmon and cook for 4–5 minutes on both sides, until cooked through.
4. Once the pasta and asparagus are cooked, drain, return the pasta to the pan and set aside the asparagus spears.
5. Add a spoonful or two of pesto to the pasta and stir through. Flake the cooked salmon into the pan. Stir well and serve with the asparagus spears (if using).

MUSHROOM AND BUTTER BEAN TOAST

Prep: 5 minutes
Cook: 15 minutes
Serves: 3, or 1 baby, 1 adult

Mushrooms aren't often an ingredient you see in many weaning books, but I'm a big fan of them and Raffy is too. This recipe came from a very random 'bish bash bosh' fridge raid and, after quickly prepping it, it was swiftly gobbled up by Raffy, meaning it's definitely a winner. This dish offers plenty of flavours and a lovely creamy texture. It's also super-easy to adapt.

1 tsp olive oil
250g mushrooms, diced
1 large knob unsalted butter
   or plant-based spread
1½ tsp plain flour
100ml milk of choice
100g butter beans, drained,
   rinsed and lightly chopped
1–2 slices bread
1 tsp fresh or dried parsley
   (well chopped if fresh)
½ tsp paprika (more if you prefer)
2 tsp yoghurt

* For baby you can blend the ingredients and offer alongside toast fingers to dip, or mash some of the mushroom and butter bean mix on to baby's toast and offer it as little finger food.

1. Heat the oil in a pan over a medium heat.
2. Add the mushrooms to the pan and cook for about 5 minutes, until browned and their liquid has evaporated.
3. Add the butter or spread and flour to make a paste.
4. Add the milk and stir well. Allow to simmer over a low heat for about 5 minutes, until the sauce has thickened. Add the butter beans and cook for 2 minutes to warm through.
5. Meanwhile, toast the bread.
6. Add the parsley, paprika and yoghurt to the pan and stir well before serving on top of the toast.

dinner

Throughout my work as a child nutritionist, I've seen time and time again the importance of sitting and eating with your baby at mealtimes; even if that's just one parent, a grandparent or a sibling, and even if it's just once a day. Eating together can really help your baby to learn eating skills, to eat more of a variety of foods and to enjoy the social side of mealtimes even more! All too often babies are simply 'fed' as we focus all our attention on feeding them and then we eat later. However, letting your little one see you eating and enjoying a wide variety of the same foods can really help them in their weaning journey and encourage them to accept and enjoy food more readily.

I like to try to encourage parents to bring baby to the table with them, as early as possible and to eat similar foods as and when they can. I understand that life gets in the way and it's not always practical to have family mealtimes every day, but even if you can eat a mini portion with baby at their mealtime and then have the rest of your main meal later on, it really can help make those mealtimes more fun and enjoyable for everyone.

These recipes are mainly for a family of four. However, it's really easy to adapt them and make more or less, depending on what you need.

FISH PIE WITH BROCCOLI MASH

Prep: 10 minutes
Cook: 35 minutes
Serves: a family of 4

This is a really easy and tasty fish pie recipe. You can easily quarter this recipe and make it in a little ramekin just for baby. However, it's often easier to make a meal for the whole family and just offer baby a portion of it.

500g potatoes, peeled and chopped
1 head of broccoli, roughly chopped
knob of unsalted butter
splash of milk of choice
300g skinless fish, such as salmon or cod,
150g frozen peas
1 x 200g tin sweetcorn, drained
juice of ½ lemon
50g Cheddar cheese, grated (optional)

For the white sauce
60g unsalted butter
60g plain flour
700ml milk of choice

✳ Mash or blend for young babies, if needed.

1. Preheat the oven to 200°C.
2. To make the mash topping, put the potatoes in a pan of boiling water and cook for 5–6 minutes, until starting to soften, then add the broccoli and cook for a further 6–8 minutes, until everything is soft and mashable.
3. Once soft, drain, add the butter and milk and mash it all together.
4. Meanwhile, make the white sauce. Melt the butter in a large pan over a medium heat, then stir in the plain flour and cook for 1 minute. Take the pan off the heat, pour in a little of the milk, then stir until blended. Gradually whisk in the remaining milk until you have a smooth sauce. Return to the heat, bring to the boil and cook for 5 minutes, stirring continually until it is nicely thickened.
5. Add the fish, peas and sweetcorn to the white sauce, squeeze in the lemon juice and mix it all up. Put this mixture into an ovenproof dish and top with the broccoli mash. Sprinkle over the Cheddar cheese (if using) and cook in the oven for 15–20 minutes, until golden on top and bubbling.

SLOW-COOKED BEEF STEW WITH GARLIC DIPPERS

Prep: 10 minutes
Cook: 3 hours
Serves: 1 baby, 2 adults

If you eat meat as a family, it's a good idea to include it in baby's diet fairly early on. That's because meat can be a little bit of an acquired taste and so babies sometimes don't accept it until they are pretty familiar with having it in their diet. Red meat is also a good source of iron (an important nutrient during weaning – see page 69), so it's fine to include it in baby's diet from around six months of age.

For the stew
1 tbsp olive oil
400g beef, well diced
1 large onion, diced
2 garlic cloves, thinly sliced
2 carrots, well chopped
1 tbsp plain flour
1 tbsp tomato puree
1 x 400g tin plum tomatoes
1 tbsp dried oregano
2 sprigs of fresh rosemary, chopped

For the garlic dippers
1 garlic clove, peeled and crushed
1 tbsp finely chopped fresh
    flat-leaf parsley
2 tbsp unsalted butter, softened
1 medium baguette, sliced
    in half lengthways

✳ You can blend the stew a little for younger babies. You can add salt and black pepper to taste to the adult portions, if you like.

1. Heat the olive oil in a large casserole dish over a high heat. Once hot, add the beef and cook for about 5 minutes, until browned all over.
2. Add the onion, garlic and carrots, then add the flour and stir to lightly coat.
3. Add the tomato puree, tinned tomatoes, oregano and rosemary with 400ml water (you can use the empty tomato tin as a guide). Give it a good mix together, breaking the tomatoes down with the back of a wooden spoon, then bring to the boil.
4. Once boiling, reduce the heat to low and cook for 2–2½ hours, until the meat is tender and the sauce is rich and thick.
5. About 15 minutes before the stew is cooked, preheat the oven to 200°C.
6. Mix the garlic and parsley with the softened butter, then spread all over the halved baguette.
7. Put the garlic-buttered baguette on to a baking tray and cook in the oven for 8–10 minutes or until golden and crusty, then slice into dippers.
8. Serve the beef stew with the garlic bread dippers for dunking!

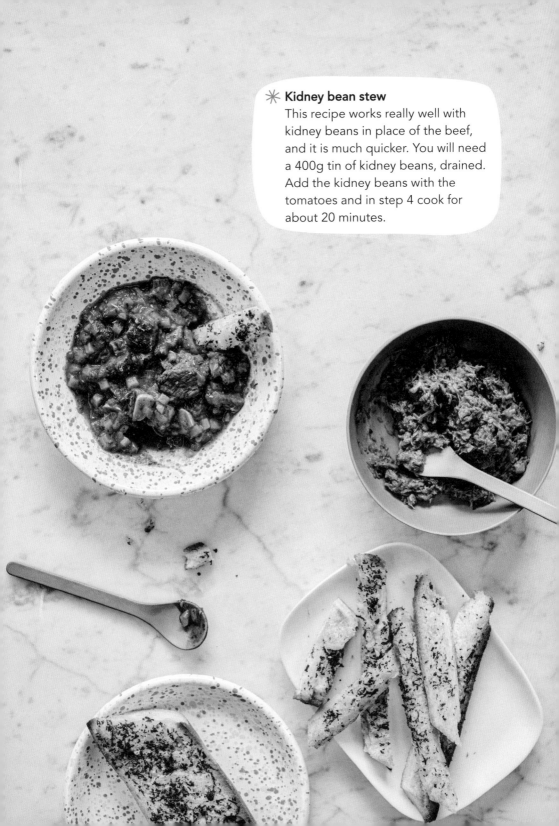

✳ Kidney bean stew

This recipe works really well with kidney beans in place of the beef, and it is much quicker. You will need a 400g tin of kidney beans, drained. Add the kidney beans with the tomatoes and in step 4 cook for about 20 minutes.

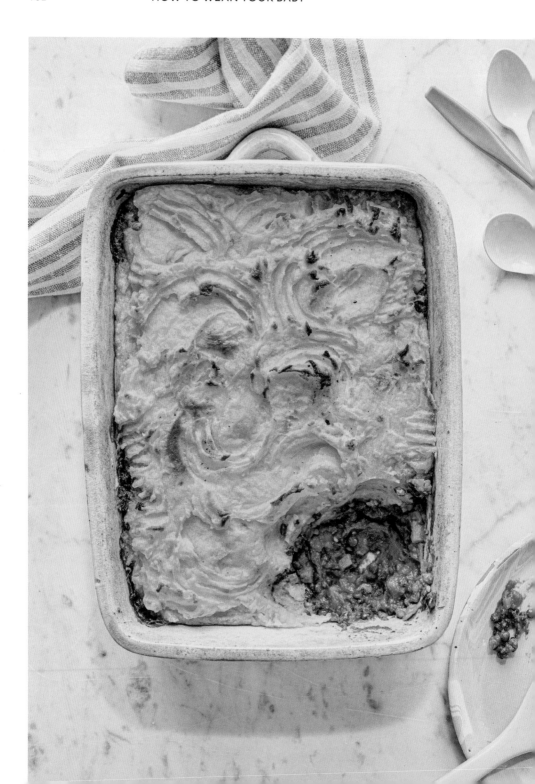

RED DRAGON PIE

Prep: 5 minutes
Cook: 1 hour
Serves: a family of 4

This is a traditional dish that I grew up with as a child. I absolutely love it and it's a great way to offer baby a really hearty and nutrient-packed meal that still tastes delicious. It's a vegetarian take on shepherd's pie, using lentils instead of mince. Using pre-cooked lentils speeds up the cooking time on this no end! If you prefer, you can slice the potatoes on top too, which helps to save time mashing. You could also swap the lentils for cooked beef mince, if you wanted to add meat.

1 tbsp oil
1 onion, finely chopped
150g carrots, peeled and finely chopped
1 tsp mixed herbs (or ¼ tsp each of basil, oregano, parsley and coriander)
2 tbsp tomato puree
100g courgette, finely chopped
250g pre-cooked puy lentils (or dried ones – cook as per packet instructions)

For the topping
500g potatoes, peeled and roughly chopped (or sliced)
25–30g unsalted butter or plant-based spread
splash of milk of your choice (if needed)

✳ For babies, mash or blend the lentil mix, if needed.
✳ This dish is really nice served with some green veggies or a side salad for the adults.

1. Heat the oil in a pan over a medium heat and cook the onions for about 5 minutes, until softened. Add the carrots and cook for a further 5 minutes.
2. Add the herbs, tomato puree and courgette and mix everything together.
3. Lastly, add the lentils with 300ml water (you could add a couple of stock ice cubes from my recipe on page 197) and bring to the boil. Simmer for 15 minutes, until the mixture is a little gloopy and the carrots are nice and soft.
4. Preheat the oven to 200°C.
5. Meanwhile, boil the potatoes for about 15 minutes. Once ready, drain, return to the pan, add the butter and mash together really well, until the potatoes are light and fluffy without lumps. Add a few splashes of milk, if needed.
6. Pour the lentil mix into an ovenproof dish and top with the mashed potato, spreading it over evenly.
7. Bake in the oven for about 30 minutes, until the potato is starting to brown nicely on top.

AVOCADO PASTA

I'm a bit of an avocado lover. It is so often used as a dip but forgotten as a perfect topping for pasta, toast, rice and potatoes!

Prep: 5 minutes
Cook: 10 minutes
Serves: a family of 4

150g penne or fusilli pasta
1 ripe avocado, destoned and
    skin removed
20g mixed nuts or pine nuts
juice of ½ lemon
2 garlic cloves
dash of olive oil

1. Cook the pasta as per the packet instructions.
2. Put all the other ingredients into a blender and blend until smooth.
3. Toss the avocado sauce with the cooked pasta and serve.

✳ If needed, you can mash or blend the pasta slightly for younger babies. Alternatively, offer as finger food pieces.

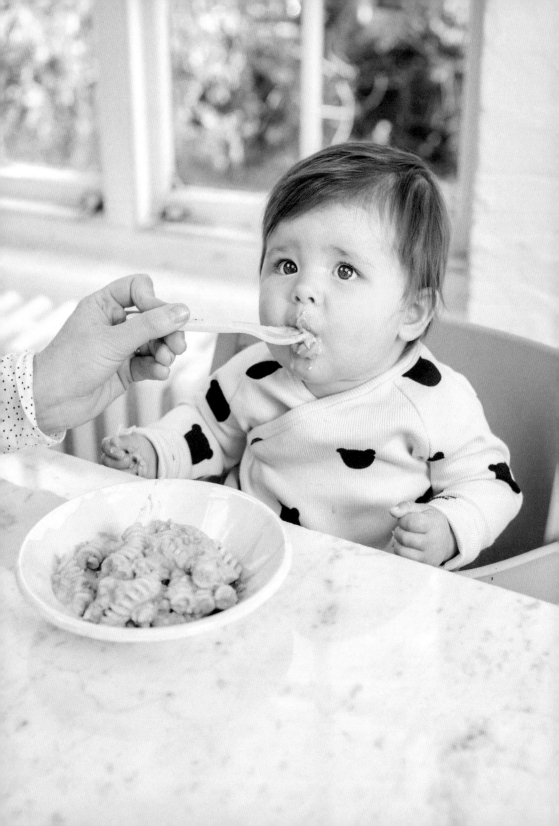

RAINBOW SPAGHETTI BOLOGNESE

This is my version of the classic recipe that just had to make it into the book! I call this 'rainbow' spag bol as it contains a great array of vegetable colours. The more colour you add to baby's diet, the better, as this means they are likely to have more variety and nutrients. In this recipe the veggies are all blended, but you don't have to, and once baby gets used to a bit more texture in their meals, you can just chop the veggies nice and small.

Prep: 10 minutes
Cook: 30 minutes
Serves: a family of 4

olive oil, for cooking
½ courgette, chopped
½ yellow pepper, chopped
2 pre-cooked beetroot, chopped
100g mushrooms, chopped
1 x 400g tin chopped tomatoes
1 onion, finely chopped
200g beef mince (or 200g tinned kidney beans, drained, mashed slightly)
1 garlic clove, finely chopped
1 tbsp tomato puree
2 tsp dried oregano
300g spaghetti
10g basil (optional)
50g Cheddar cheese, grated (optional)

✳ You can mash or blend this further, if needed for younger babies, or simply chop the spaghetti a little and let baby dig in!

1. Heat a drizzle of olive oil in a pan over a medium-high heat and cook the courgette, pepper, beetroot and mushrooms for about 5 minutes, until softened.
2. Once softened, transfer the cooked vegetables to a food processor, add the tomatoes and blend until smooth.
3. Reusing the pan, heat a little more olive oil over a medium heat then add the onion and beef mince (or kidney beans) and cook for about 10 minutes, until the beef has browned all over.
4. Add the garlic and cook for a further minute. Add the tomato puree, oregano and the veg sauce from the blender. Stir together and bring to the boil.
5. Once boiling, reduce to a simmer and cook for 10 minutes, until reduced and the flavours have all come together. Meanwhile, cook the spaghetti following the packet instructions (about 10 minutes).
6. Serve the sauce over the spaghetti and sprinkle with chopped basil and grated cheese (if using).

OVEN-BAKED FALAFEL WRAPS

Prep: 10 minutes
Cook: 30 minutes
Serves: 1 baby, 1 adult

These falafel make perfect little savoury snacks on their own or can be served with some veggie sticks and a dollop of hummus for a light meal, or made into wraps. Younger babies can just have torn up bits of wrap with finger food pieces of falafel and a hummus dip, but as your baby develops their skills with self-feeding you can advance to more of a wrap shape.

For the falafel (makes 10 falafel)
1 x 400g tin chickpeas,
    drained and rinsed
1 small red onion, chopped
10g flat-leaf parsley, chopped
1 tsp ground cumin
1 tsp ground coriander
1 tbsp plain flour
juice of ½ lemon
olive oil, for cooking

For the wraps
1 tortilla wrap
1 tbsp Chickpea Dip (see page 193)
1 pre-cooked beetroot, thinly sliced
½ carrot, peeled and finely grated
    (for baby)

✳ For babies who are good with textures, you can slice these wraps once rolled widthways to offer as little finger foods. For younger babies, offer the falafel with some torn-up wrap, pieces of cooked beetroot and Chickpea Dip.

1. Preheat the oven to 200°C.
2. Pat the chickpeas dry with kitchen paper (they don't need to be completely dry but this helps the falafel hold together). Put the chickpeas in a food processor with the red onion, parsley, cumin and coriander.
3. Blitz until smooth, then add the flour and lemon juice and blitz again until all mixed together.
4. Drizzle a baking tray with a little olive oil (to stop the falafel from sticking). Shape the mixture into about 10 balls and put them on the tray. The mixture should feel like a sticky dough, but if they're not sticking together well add a little extra flour.
5. Drizzle the falafel with a little olive oil then bake for 25–30 minutes or until golden and crisp, turning halfway through.
6. While the falafel are cooking, prepare your wrap. Spread with a spoonful of Chickpea Dip then top with the beetroot and carrot. Repeat if you are making more.
7. Once the falafel are cooked, add them to the wraps and fold them up!

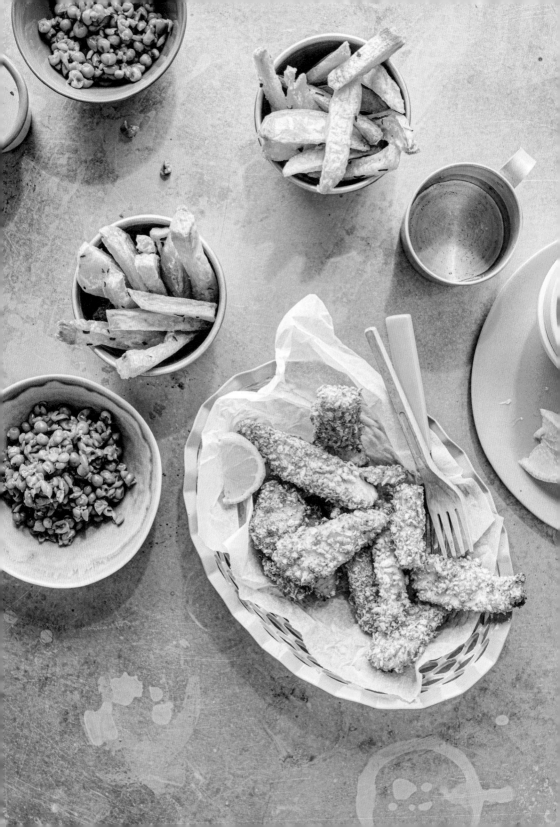

WITCH AND CHIPS

Prep: 15 minutes
Cook: 40 minutes
Serves: a family of 4

Many kids love takeaway fish and chips, but it's actually pretty easy to recreate this dish at home. It has this name in our house due to the Julia Donaldson books; anyone else got a *Room on the Broom* fan? This recipe also means you can make an unsalted version for baby without too much saturated fat. It's a bit messy to make, but it's definitely worth it.

3 large baking potatoes, scrubbed or peeled and chopped into finger-shaped chips
2–3 tbsp olive oil
2 sprigs of fresh rosemary, chopped
450g white fish, deboned, deskinned and chopped into rough chunks or finger-shaped strips
100g breadcrumbs (about 2 slices bread, blended into breadcrumbs)
zest of ½ lemon
1 tsp paprika
1 free-range egg
120g frozen peas

✳ For younger babies you can mash or chop as needed, or offer as fish and chip finger foods. Mash the peas a little for younger babies.

1. Put the potatoes into a pan of water and boil for 6–8 minutes.
2. Preheat the oven to 200°C. Put the olive oil in a roasting tin and place in the oven. Line a baking tray with greaseproof paper. Once the potatoes are softened, add them to the heated roasting tin along with the sprigs of rosemary and cook in the oven for about 30 minutes, until browning nicely.
3. Meanwhile, put the breadcrumbs in a bowl and add the lemon zest and paprika. Mix well and spread out on a flat plate.
4. Break the egg into a shallow bowl and beat.
5. Dip the fish in the egg mixture, shake off any excess and then dip it in the breadcrumbs. Make sure the fish is well covered with breadcrumbs (you might need to press the breadcrumbs down on either side of the fish).
6. Pop the breadcrumbed fish on the lined baking tray and add to the oven for about 20 minutes.
7. Meanwhile, boil the peas for 5 minutes.
8. Once ready, serve the fish and chips together with the peas.

MEXICAN STUFFED JACKETS

Prep: 20 minutes
Cook: 35 minutes
Serves: a family of 4

It's such a good idea to get baby used to different culinary tastes and flavours in their diet. We love experimenting with new foods and flavours for Raffy, especially when travelling or on holiday. It's great to get them out of their food comfort zone a little sometimes, even from a young age. However, there is no reason why you can't bring some of those culinary tastes into your own home. This Mexican dish is so flexible – simply choose two or three of your favourite fillings and fill your potato as you like. Finish with the sour cream and a sprinkling of cheese!

---

4 sweet potatoes
4 tbsp sour cream
grated cheese, to serve

✳ For baby you can simply mash the sweet potato insides with some of the fillings. Mash/blend the dips further as needed.

1. Preheat the oven to 200°C.
2. Pierce the potatoes and bake in the oven for 30–35 minutes.
3. Once cooked, open out the sweet potato jackets and top with a few spoons of each of the toppings opposite, along with a little sour cream and a sprinkling of cheese.

CHICKEN AND BLACK BEAN DIP

1 tsp olive oil
1 red onion, finely chopped
2 chicken breasts
1 garlic clove, finely chopped
1 tbsp tomato puree
2 tsp smoked paprika
2 tsp ground cumin
1 x 400g tin black beans,
    drained and rinsed

1. Heat the olive oil in a pan over a medium heat and cook the red onion for about 5 minutes.
2. Add the chicken breasts and cook for 3 minutes on each side until browned (stir the onions around so they don't burn!).
3. Add the garlic, tomato puree, smoked paprika and cumin and cook for another minute.
4. Add the beans plus half a tinful of cold water (about 200ml), bring to the boil over a high heat, then reduce to a simmer with the pan lid on for 10–15 minutes, until the chicken is cooked through and the sauce has thickened.
5. Once the chicken is cooked, shred it apart using two forks.
6. Roughly mash the beans with a fork and mix everything together.

✳ This dish can easily be made without the chicken, if you don't eat meat.
✳ Mash further or blend a little for baby, if needed

SWEETCORN SALSA

1 x 200g tin sweetcorn, drained
1 spring onion/shallot, thinly sliced
a small handful of coriander,
    roughly chopped
juice of ½ lime

1. Mix all ingredients together in a bowl.
2. Blend half or all of the mixture for just a few seconds. If just doing half, mix together again at the end.

GUACAMOLE

2 ripe avocados, destoned, skin
    removed, mashed well with a fork
1 tbsp extra virgin olive oil
1 garlic clove, finely chopped or crushed
a small handful of coriander, very
    finely chopped
juice of ½ lime

1. Put all the ingredients into a bowl and mix well.

TOMATO SALSA

150g tomatoes (or 1 medium beef
    tomato), well chopped
½ red onion, finely chopped
a drizzle of extra virgin olive oil

1. Mash the chopped tomato slightly with a fork.
2. Put the tomato and onion in a bowl and drizzle over a little olive oil.

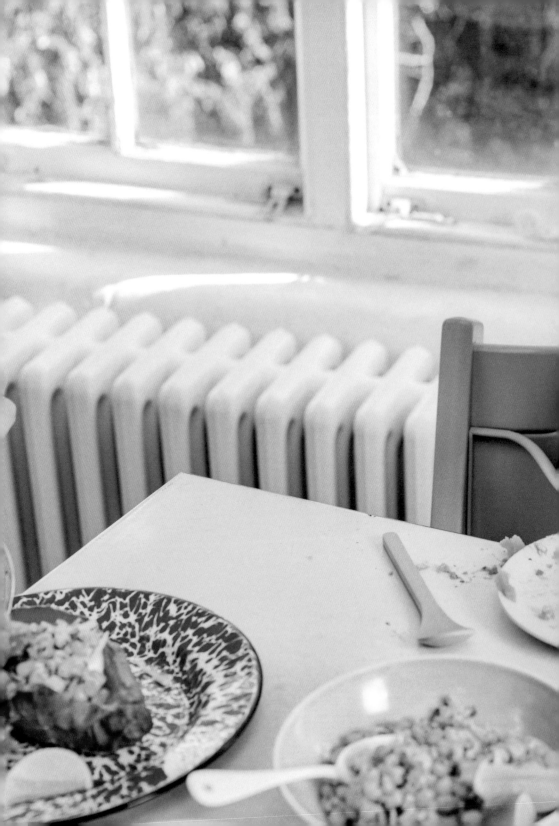

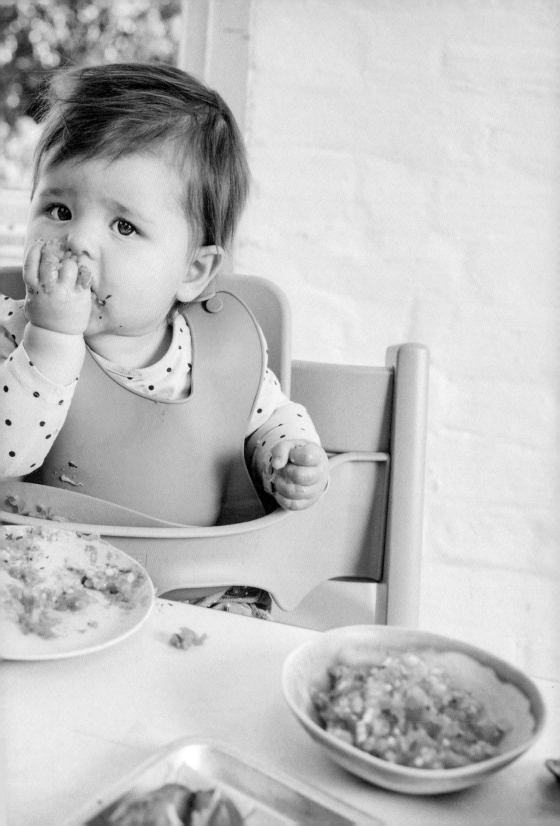

BABY'S FIRST CURRY

I love this recipe as it's full of nutritious ingredients and is really simple to put together. This recipe uses coconut milk to add some delicious creaminess to the curry. You can experiment a little more with the flavours and spices used, if you wish.

Prep: 5 minutes
Cook: 40 minutes
Serves: 1 baby, 2 adults

---

1 tbsp olive oil
1–2 tsp garam masala
1 tsp turmeric
a pinch of garlic granules
1 heaped tsp tomato puree
200g sweet potato, peeled and diced
1 chicken breast, chopped or ½ x 400g tin chickpeas, drained and rinsed
½ x 400ml tin coconut milk
170g cauliflower, chopped into small manageable pieces for baby
80g frozen peas

✳ Mash the curry well for younger babies, if needed, and serve with rice or some bread fingers to dip.

1. Heat the oil in a large pan over a medium heat and add the garam masala, turmeric and garlic granules. Stir well and cook for a few minutes.
2. Add the tomato puree and stir well until you've made a paste, then add the sweet potato and chicken and stir well until both are fully coated.
3. Add the coconut milk and 80ml water, then bring to the boil before turning the heat down to a simmer. Cook for 15 minutes.
4. Add the cauliflower and stir for a few minutes (add the chickpeas now if using instead of chicken) and cook for a further 5–10 minutes – add a few splashes of water at this stage if the sauce looks too thick.
5. Add the peas and cook for a further 5 minutes.
6. Serve with rice or some warm flatbread (see page 193).

BABY'S FIRST BURGER

Prep: 5 minutes
Cook: 10–15 minutes
Makes: 8 mini burgers or 1 large burger and 2–3 mini burgers

I didn't feel this book would be complete without making a recipe for baby's first burger. Don't worry there is a veggie version on page 176! Burgers don't have to be the greasy ones you find at takeaways – they can be perfectly healthy options for baby to have in their diet as well as super-simple to make.

300g beef/turkey mince
2 spring onions, well chopped
½ tsp garlic powder or 1 garlic
    clove, crushed
1 free-range egg, beaten
1 tsp paprika
1 tsp cumin
1 tbsp olive oil, for frying
Tomato Salsa (see page 171) and
    mini burger buns, to serve

1. Put all the ingredients (except the olive oil) into a bowl and mix together with your hands.
2. Form the mixture into mini burger shapes (8 mini, or 1 large and 2–3 mini). Heat the oil in a pan over a medium heat and fry the burgers for about 4 minutes on each side.
3. Serve with Tomato Salsa in mini burger buns or warmed pitta breads, and a side of greens.

✳ Chop into little finger-shaped pieces for young babies and serve with some tomato fingers and a mini bun.

BABY'S FIRST VEGAN BURGER

Prep: 10 minutes
Cook: 20 minutes
Makes: 6 mini burgers

For this recipe I took inspiration from my good friend Joe Wicks, who makes a fantastic vegan bean burger which all goes in one bowl and you squidge it together with your hands! It's such a quick win for a BBQ or a little dinner for you and baby! This one goes really well with Tomato Salsa (see page 171) and a little Chickpea Dip (see page 193).

½ x 400g tin chickpeas, drained and mashed well
½ x 400g tin black beans, drained
2 spring onions, finely chopped
½ tsp garlic powder or 1 garlic clove, finely chopped or crushed
1 tsp cumin
1 tsp paprika
1 tbsp plain flour (or use a gluten-free alternative)
olive oil, for cooking
Tomato Salsa (see page 171), Chickpea Dip (see page 193) and burger buns

✳ Offer as finger food burgers for younger babies alongside some sliced beef tomatoes and bread fingers.

1. Preheat the oven to 200°C. Line a baking tray with greaseproof paper.
2. Put all the ingredients (aside from the oil) in a bowl and mix really well with your hands. Crush the ingredients together really well – it might take a little time and effort to get them really well mixed.
3. Shape the mixture into 6 small burger shapes and sprinkle each with a little oil. Place on the lined baking tray and bake in the oven for 20 minutes (turn them halfway through).
4. Serve with Tomato Salsa and Chickpea Dip in mini burger buns or warmed pitta breads, and a side of greens.

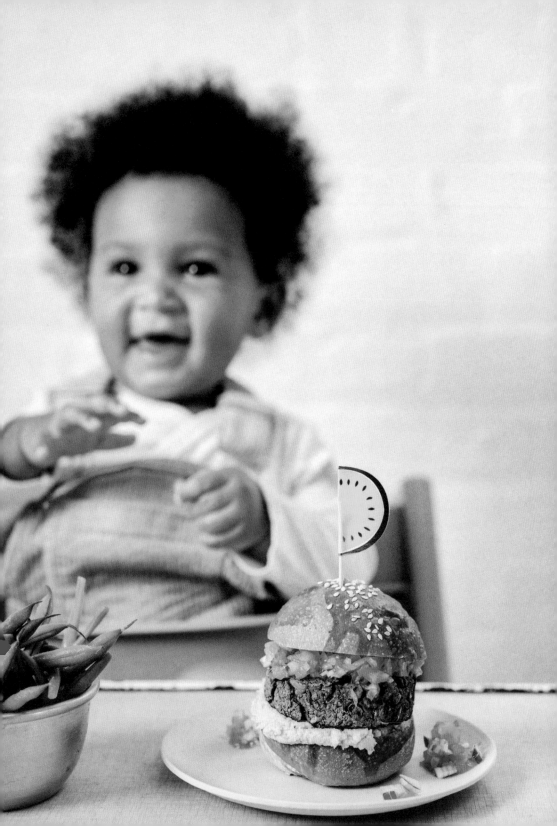

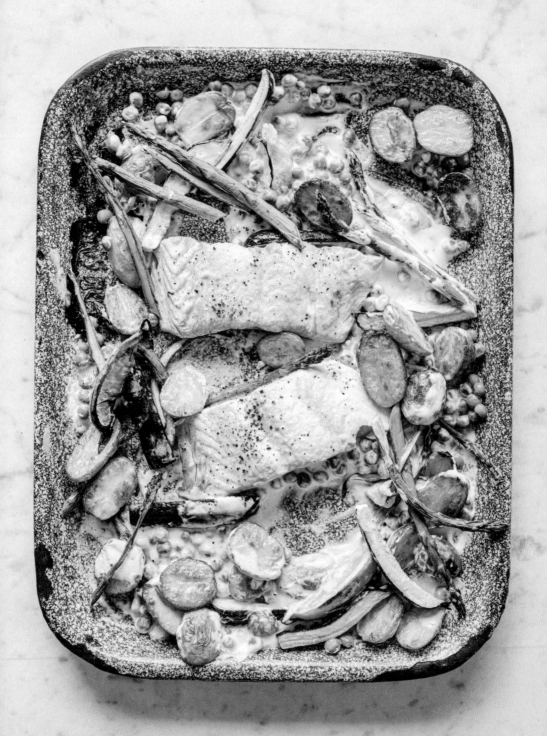

CREAMY LEMONY SALMON BAKE

Prep: 5 minutes
Cook: 35 minutes
Serves: 1 baby, 2 adults

This is such a lovely dish to offer to baby and is a really simple way to cook a healthy family meal. I love this one as a quick Sunday lunch for the whole family and have made it on a number of occasions! If you want to make this for a family of four, just add another fillet of salmon and a few extra veggies.

300g baby new potatoes, halved
  or in sticks
1 courgette, cut into sticks
a drizzle of olive oil
100g full-fat soft cheese
1 lemon
125g asparagus, woody ends
  removed, chopped in half
2 salmon fillets
100g frozen peas

※ For young babies you can blend or mash the veggies with some of the sauce and serve alongside strips of the baked salmon. Or offer all as little finger foods for baby to self-feed.

1. Preheat the oven to 200°C.
2. Put the new potatoes and courgette in a baking tray, drizzle over the olive oil and cook for 15–20 minutes, until starting to soften and brown. For younger babies, remove the skin from some of the potatoes and courgettes, when cooled.
3. Whisk together the cream cheese with 200ml boiling water until smooth, then squeeze in the juice of half the lemon and cut the other half into 2 wedges.
4. Add the asparagus and lemon wedges to the tray, then lay the salmon fillets (skin-side up) on top and return to the oven for another 10 minutes, until the salmon is almost cooked.
5. Add the frozen peas then drizzle the lemony cream cheese mixture all over (make sure all the peas are covered in liquid so they cook properly!).
6. Cook for a final 5 minutes then serve, spooning the creamy sauce all over. Make sure you remove the salmon skin before serving this to baby.

TRAFFIC LIGHT LASAGNE

Prep: 10 minutes
Cook: 1 hour
Serves: a family of 4

I'm a bit of a fan of Italian food and I love making lasagne, but when cooking for baby it can be a bit time-consuming! I've made this one with my cheat's version of béchamel sauce, to speed things up. I've also used lots of extra flavours to really give this dinner a kick. If you prefer standard béchamel simply use the sauce from my Mac and Cheese on page 152, but I think this works just as well!

For the cheat's béchamel
250g crème fraîche
30g cheese, grated, plus extra
    to top the lasagne
4 tbsp hot water
a large pinch of nutmeg

For the tomato sauce
1 tbsp olive oil
1 red onion, diced
1–2 garlic cloves, chopped
1 red pepper, well chopped
1 tbsp tomato puree
2 tsp mixed herbs
1 x 400g tin chopped tomatoes, drained
1 x 400g tin lentils, including the water
1 x 200g tin sweetcorn, drained

For the layers
100g fresh spinach
9–10 dried lasagne sheets

✳ Chop or mash the lasagne well for baby, if needed.

1. To make the cheat's béchamel, put the crème fraiche, cheese, hot water and nutmeg in a bowl. Stir together well and leave to one side.
2. To make the tomato sauce, heat the olive oil in a pan over a medium heat then add the red onion. Cook for 5 minutes, then add the garlic and cook for about 5 minutes, until softened.
3. Add the red pepper, tomato puree, mixed herbs, tomatoes and lentils (including the water), and cook over a medium heat for about 10 minutes, stirring every now and then.
4. Preheat the oven to 200°C.
5. Add the sweetcorn to the lentil mixture and cook for another 5 minutes. Remove from the heat (you can blend the mixture now if you think it's needed for younger babies).
6. Now start layering your lasagne, following the steps opposite.
7. Cook in the oven for 20–30 minutes, until the top starts to brown and the lasagne starts to bubble a little.

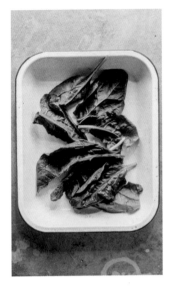

1. Start with a scattering of spinach on the bottom of an ovenproof dish.

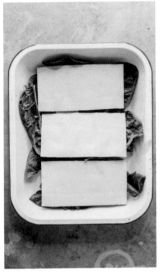

2. Cover the spinach with lasagne sheets.

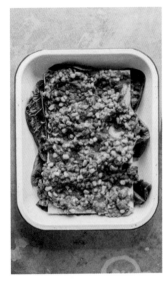

3. Add half the lentil sauce.

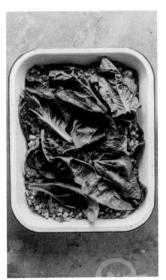

4. Add more spinach.

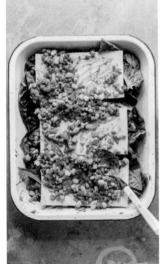

5. Add more lasagne sheets and the rest of the lentil sauce.

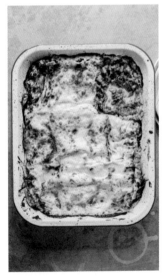

6. Finally, add more lasagne sheets, pour over the béchamel sauce and sprinkle with grated cheese.

THAI GREEN CURRY

Prep: 5 minutes
Cook: 10 minutes (plus rice cooking time)
Serves: a family of 4

Another flavour-packed dish to help develop baby's taste buds! Although there are a fair few ingredients in this dish, it is a great way to make a quick Thai curry sauce. Prep the veg with your baby in mind – in batons for them to hold as finger foods or chopped small to add texture to the meal.

brown rice, to serve

For the paste
25g fresh coriander, roughly chopped
1 lemongrass stalk, outer stalk removed, roughly chopped
1 shallot, roughly chopped
2 garlic cloves, roughly chopped
thumb-sized piece of fresh root ginger, peeled and chopped
juice of ½ lime
1 tsp ground cumin
1 tbsp vegetable oil

For the curry
100g baby corn, halved lengthways
100g green beans, halved
100g mangetout
1 x 400ml tin full-fat coconut milk
300g raw king prawns or 280g extra-firm tofu, drained and cut into small cubes

1. Cook the brown rice as per the packet instructions.
2. To make the paste, put the coriander, lemongrass, shallot, garlic and ginger into a food processor and blitz until smooth.
3. Squeeze in the lime juice, add the ground cumin and vegetable oil and mix it all together.
4. Tip the paste into a non-stick frying pan or wok and cook over a high heat for 2–3 minutes, until sizzling and fragrant.
5. Add the baby corn, green beans and mangetout and stir to coat them in the paste.
6. Add the coconut milk, prawns or tofu and cook for 4–5 minutes or until the vegetables are softened and the prawns are cooked through and pink.
7. Serve with brown rice and tuck in!

✳ This can be served to baby as finger food vegetable sticks with the curry sauce and rice, or blend the recipe up a little before serving.

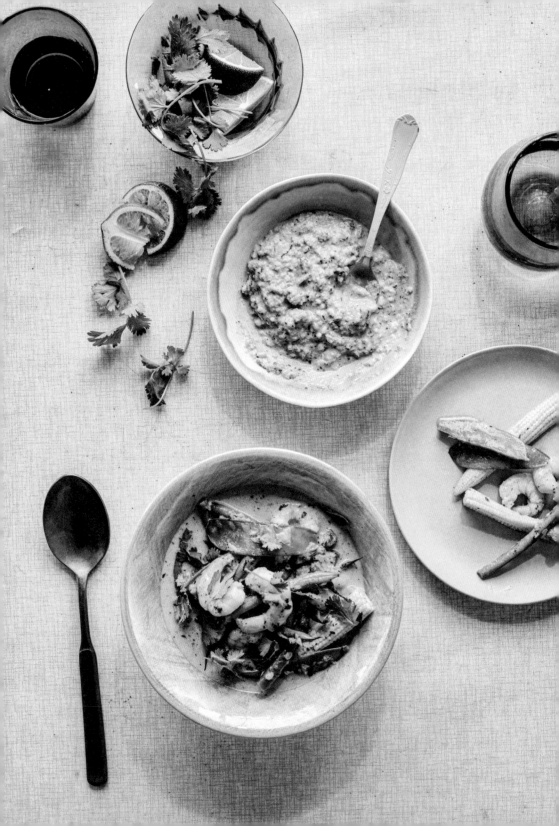

SUPER EASY, VEG-PACKED CHILLI

Prep: 10 minutes
Cook: 45 minutes
Serves: a family of 4

Everyone loves a chilli, and it's a great way to get your little one used to some new flavours in their foods. Using actual chilli might be all right for older children, but it's best not to add very hot spices to baby's food; paprika and cumin give this a lovely flavour. If you want to add more in the way of spice and flavours as your baby experiments, that's great. Additionally, feel free to add a little more into your own dish at the end.

---

1 tbsp olive oil
1 red onion, diced
1 tsp paprika
1 tsp cumin
½ tsp chilli (for babies who are experienced with flavours, optional)
1 tbsp tomato puree
1 medium sweet potato, peeled and chopped into small pieces
1 red pepper, roughly chopped
100g mushrooms, roughly chopped
1 x 400g tin chopped tomatoes
1 x 400g tin kidney beans, drained and rinsed
Brown rice or pitta breads, yoghurt or guacamole, to serve (optional)

1. Heat the oil in a pan over a medium heat and cook the onion for about 5 minutes, then add the paprika, cumin, chilli (if using), tomato puree, sweet potato, pepper and mushrooms. Stir well and cook for 5 minutes.
2. Add the tinned tomatoes and kidney beans and bring to a simmer.
3. Cook the chilli with the lid on for 20–25 minutes before removing the lid and then cooking for another 10 minutes.
4. You can eat this as it is or serve with some brown rice or pitta breads and a nice dollop of yoghurt. You could also try serving with some guacamole on the side (see page 171).

✳ For younger babies you can blend or roughly mash the chilli, as needed, adding a splash of water if needed.

Finger foods, light bites and puds

Here is the really fun part of the recipe section! In the following pages you'll find my ideas for little finger foods for baby to try and practise their skills on, as well as some lighter lunches and meal ideas if you and baby are eating on the go, or just need something small. It's not always practical to create more substantial meals and, let's face it, there are always going to be plenty of days when you just want a quick-fix option for baby's lunchtime!

Sometimes it can be useful to offer baby puddings as a little nutrient top-up after their main meal or lunch. It can be fun every now and then to have pudding together, and these recipes prove that pudding doesn't have to be sweet and sugary.

SPINACH AND CHEDDAR MUFFINS

These mini muffins are a perfect breakfast muffin or on-the-go snack. You can also team them with some veggie sticks and dips and offer as a light lunch. I've made these for a few parties and they always go down really well, especially when they are warm out of the oven.

Prep: 10 minutes
Cook: 25 minutes
Makes: 12 muffins

80g spinach
2 free-range eggs
100ml milk of choice
50g unsalted butter, melted,
    plus extra for greasing
150g self-raising flour
120g Cheddar cheese, grated
3 spring onions, thinly sliced

1. Preheat the oven to 200°C. Line a 12-hole muffin tray with cases or grease the holes with a little butter.
2. Put the spinach in a colander in the sink and pour a kettleful of boiling water over it until it's all wilted. Rinse the wilted spinach with cold water until it is cool enough to handle then squeeze out as much of the water as possible and pat it dry with kitchen paper. Once it is as dry as you can get it, roughly chop.
3. Beat the eggs in a large bowl then add the milk and melted butter and combine. Add the flour, cheese, spring onions and chopped wilted spinach and mix until evenly distributed.
4. Divide the batter between the muffin cases and cook for 15–20 minutes, until golden and a skewer comes out clean.

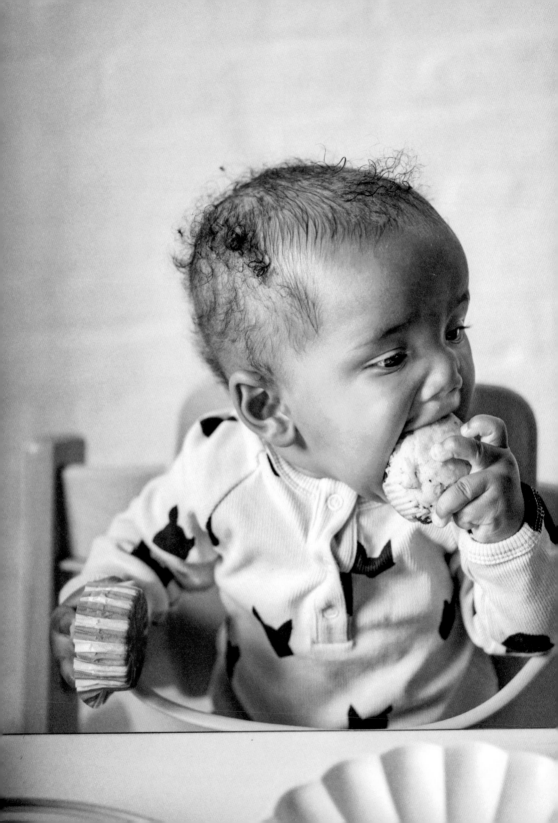

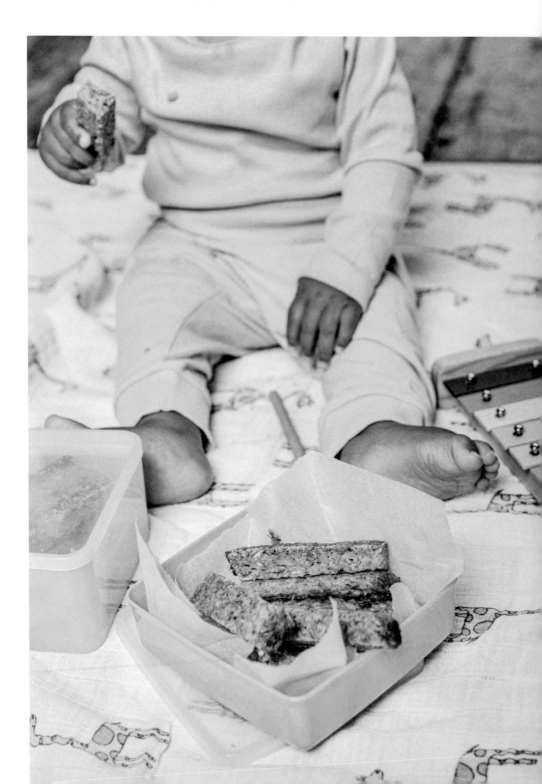

CARROT OAT BARS

Prep: 5 minutes
Cook: 20 minutes
Makes: 8–10 bars

Raffy loved these when I was experimenting with recipes for this book, so they had to go in. They are really simple and a great way to get some extra veg into your baby or toddler's diet.

olive oil or butter, to grease
½ carrot, peeled and grated
½ small apple, peeled and grated
2 bananas, mashed
1 tbsp smooth, 100 per cent almond butter
150g oats

1. Preheat the oven to 200°C. Lightly grease a baking tray.
2. Add all the ingredients to a large bowl and mix together with your hands or a spoon.
3. Press the mixture into the greased baking tray.
4. Bake in the oven for 20 minutes. Leave to cool before cutting into 8–10 bars.

✳ These make perfect little finger food bars for any age.

CHEESE BISCUITS

Prep: 5 minutes
Cook: 10 minutes
Makes: about 10 biscuits

These are such a quick, simple and tasty option for babies and toddlers. If your baby is under one, you could serve these with some veggie sticks or offer as a snack for older children.

50g ground almonds
50g cheese, finely grated
a few pinches of dried basil or oregano

1. Preheat the oven to 200°C. Line a baking tray with greaseproof paper.
2. Put the ingredients in a bowl and mix together. Using a metal spoon, press the mixture hard into a spoon, making round biscuit shapes. Slide the mixture off the spoon on to the baking tray and repeat until you have about 10 biscuits.
3. Bake for about 10 minutes, until nicely browned.
4. Remove from the oven and allow to cool and harden before serving.

BABY'S FIRST ICE CREAM

Prep: 5 minutes
Serves: 4

On a hot day offering your little one an ice cream is a perfect way to keep them cool and hydrated. It can take a while for babies to get used to the coldness of ice cream, but this recipe is a great first ice cream taste, with plenty of nutrients and not too sweet.

225g frozen berries (I like the forest fruits mixtures)
40g frozen spinach (optional)
150g yoghurt

1. Add all the ingredients to a blender and blend until smooth.
2. Serve a scoop in a bowl straight away, or pop into ice lolly moulds and freeze.

BABY'S FIRST OMELETTE

Prep: 5 minutes
Cook: 5 minutes
Serves: 1–2 babies

Omelettes are just such a quick and easy win as a light bite for baby – either as a lunch or breakfast. You can vary what you add to omelettes, or make it plain (no veg) if you're worried initially about the lumpy bits.

olive oil, for cooking
1 tbsp frozen veggies, such as peas, carrots and broccoli
1 free-range egg
a pinch of oregano
a little cheese, grated (optional)

1. Heat the oil in a frying pan over a medium heat. Add the veggies and fry for a few of minutes, until defrosted and softened.
2. In a bowl, whisk the egg with the oregano and then add to the frying pan with the softened veg.
3. Cook for 2–3 minutes before adding the cheese (if using) and allow it to melt. Make sure the eggs are cooked all the way through before turning out on to a plate.

✳ Serve in strips for baby to feed themselves along with some bread or toast fingers.

CHICKPEA FLATBREAD

Prep: 2 minutes
Cook: 10 minutes
Makes: 4 flatbreads

This is such an easy way to make bread at home. They look a little like pancakes, but have a very different taste and are also gluten-free for those families or babies who can't have gluten!

125g chickpea (gram) flour
½ tsp bicarbonate of soda
a drizzle of olive oil, for cooking

1. Put the chickpea flour and bicarbonate of soda in a large bowl.
2. Whisk in 200ml cold water until smooth to form a batter.
3. Heat the olive oil in a large non-stick pan over a medium heat. Once hot, add a ladleful of the batter and swirl it around the pan, using the back of the ladle to gently push the mixture out to form a neat circle.
4. Cook for 2–3 minutes, until set and starting to brown and then flip, cooking the other side for a further minute until golden brown. Repeat with the rest of the batter.

✳ Serve in finger food strips for baby. These flatbreads go well with soups, dips or as an alternative to the Garlic Bread Dippers on page 160.

ONE DIP,
FOUR WAYS

Prep: 2–40 minutes
Makes: 4–8 servings each dip

This was the first recipe I created for this book. I had the idea of having one standard base and showing ways to change it up so you can offer baby a variety of different dip flavours. All of these start with one simple base and you just adapt the flavours as you and your family need. These are perfect for a party too!

FOR THE BASE

1 tbsp olive oil
1 tbsp lemon juice
1 tbsp tahini

✳ Tahini is sesame seed paste, so if your baby hasn't had it before, offer it as per the allergy recommendations on page 56.

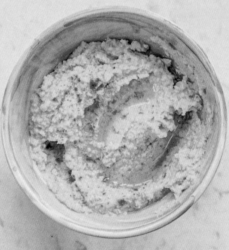

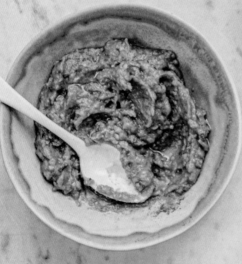

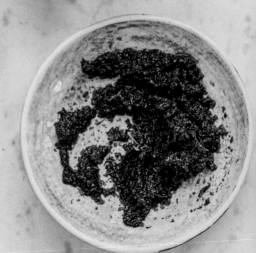

AUBERGINE DIP

1 aubergine
a few pinches of smoked paprika
a drizzle of olive oil

1. Preheat the oven to 200°C.
2. Cut the aubergine in half lengthways
   and score the middle of the flesh.
   Rub the paprika and olive oil into
   the flesh and bake in the oven for
   30–40 minutes.
3. Once cooked, scrape the flesh out
   and discard the skin. Put the flesh into
   a blender with the rest of the base
   ingredients and blend until well mixed.

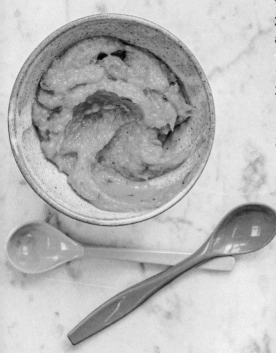

CHICKPEA DIP (HUMMUS)

1 x 400g tin chickpeas, drained
  and rinsed
1 garlic clove, crushed
a few pinches of paprika, to taste
a little olive oil, to blend

1. Put all the ingredients into a blender
   with the base ingredients and blend until
   smooth. Add olive oil as needed until you
   get your desired texture/consistency.

BUTTERNUT SQUASH DIP

½ butternut squash, seeds removed
2 sprigs of sage, leaves picked
a little olive oil, for blending

1. Preheat the oven to 200°C.
2. Place the butternut squash on a baking
   tray and roast in the oven for 30–40
   minutes.
3. Once cooked, scoop out the middle and
   add it to a blender with the sage and
   the rest of the base ingredients. Add
   olive oil as needed and blend until you
   get your desired texture/consistency.

BEETROOT DIP

2 large cooked beetroot, skins removed
2 sprigs of dill

1. Put the beetroot and dill in a blender
   with the base ingredients and blend
   until smooth and well mixed.

MY FIRST BIRTHDAY CAKE AKA FRUIT TOWER

If you're looking for the ideal birthday cake for your little one but you're not quite ready for them to have a slice of standard cake, this might just be the one for you. We offered this to Raffy on his first birthday and you should have seen his face light up. He really enjoyed munching on the squashed berries and slices of his fruit tower!

Prep: 15 minutes
Serves: 8

1 pineapple, peeled
1 watermelon, peeled
1 melon, peeled
blueberries, strawberries, grapes
   and raspberries, to decorate

✳Please remember that young babies will need to have blueberries and grapes chopped well before serving.

1. Use a knife to cut 2cm-thick circles out of the pineapple, watermelon and melon. Gradually make each of the circles you create smaller so that you can stack them on top of one another, making a tower.
2. Use 1 or 2 kebab sticks to push down through the circles to keep them in place.
3. Poke 4 more sticks into the top of the tower and slide on a variety of berries.
4. Throw a few more chopped berries around the bottom of the cake, and add a candle to finish off the decoration!

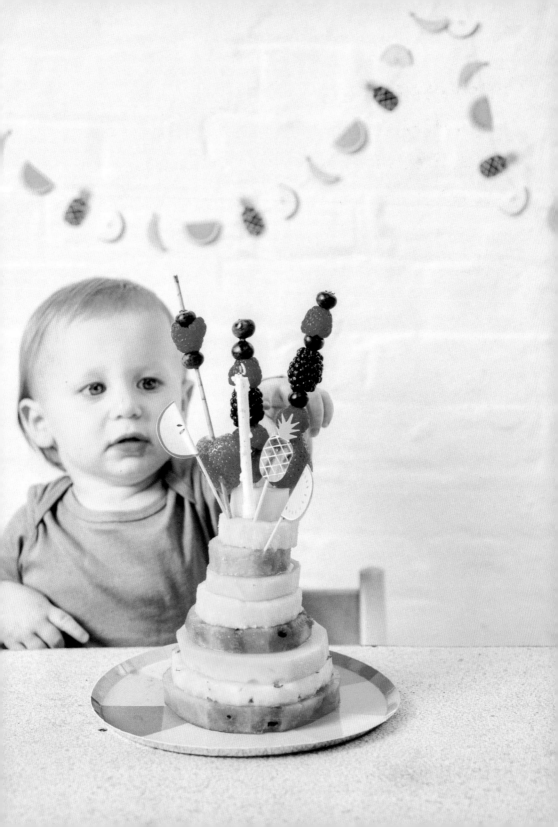

LEFTOVER VEG MUFFINS

Prep: 5 minutes
Cook: 20 minutes
Makes: 5–6 muffins

These muffins are a great quick and easy, on-the-go snack or a light meal option. They are also a perfect way of using up any veg that is left over from when shopping for the other recipes in this book.

olive oil or butter, to grease
3 large free-range eggs
a grind of black pepper (optional)
100g leftover veg (such as tomatoes, onions, spinach, peppers, sweetcorn, carrots or celery), chopped really small
15g Cheddar cheese, grated (optional)

1. Preheat the oven to 200°C. Line a 6-hole muffin tray with six cases or grease the holes with a little olive oil or butter.
2. Whisk the eggs, adding a little grind of black pepper (if using) and pour the mixture up to halfway in each of the muffin holes.
3. Fill the rest of the holes with the chopped vegetables. Top each with a sprinkling of grated cheese (if using).
4. Bake in the oven for 15–20 minutes, until golden on top.
5. Serve as a snack or as part of a meal with some vegetable sticks and bread, if you like.

RHUBARB CRUMBLE

Prep: 10 minutes
Cook: 30 minutes
Serves: a family of 4

This is such a simple way to make crumble, and it's perfect for young ones as there are lots of different flavours in it and no added sugar!

300g rhubarb, roughly chopped
2 bananas, mashed
a large pinch of ground ginger
½ lemon
75g rolled oats
75g plain flour
60g unsalted butter or plant-based spread
a large pinch of cinnamon
a large pinch of nutmeg
yoghurt, to serve (optional)

1. Preheat the oven to 200°C.
2. Steam the rhubarb for about 8 minutes, until soft and ready to eat.
3. Put the rhubarb in a baking dish and add the bananas, ginger and a few squeezes of lemon juice. Mix well.
4. Put the oats, flour, butter or spread, cinnamon and nutmeg into a bowl, then rub it together with your fingers until you make a crumble topping.
5. Scatter the crumble topping over the rhubarb mixture and add a few extra squeezes of lemon juice.
6. Bake in the oven for about 20 minutes or until the oats on top are golden brown.
7. Serve with a dollop of yoghurt.

VEGGIE STOCK RECIPE

Prep: 5 minutes
Cook: 1 hour 5 minutes
Makes: about 800 ml or 4 ice-cube trays of frozen stock

So many parents ask about stock cubes, but the truth is that even the low-salt ones still contain some added salt, which isn't ideal when cooking for younger babies. This is a fab recipe that you can make in bulk, freeze in ice-cube trays and pop out to add to recipes throughout this book for a little extra flavour here and there.

2 tbsp olive oil
2 large carrots, peeled and grated
2 celery sticks, grated
1 large onion, thinly sliced
1 large garlic clove, halved
4–5 sprigs of fresh thyme
2 sprigs fresh of rosemary
3 bay leaves
a few grinds of black pepper
1 tsp tomato puree
2g dried porcini mushrooms

1. Heat the olive oil in a pan over a medium heat and add the carrots, celery, onion and garlic. Cook for about 5 minutes, until softened.
2. Add the thyme, rosemary, bay leaves, black pepper, tomato puree and mushrooms and cover with 1 litre boiling water from the kettle.
3. Bring to the boil and simmer for 1 hour. Allow to sit and cool for 30 minutes.
4. Drain the liquid to remove most of the vegetables and herbs, and then squeeze out this mixture, using a muslin cloth or tea towel to get as much flavour and nutrients into the stock liquid.
5. Freeze in ice-cube trays and pop out frozen cubes of stock when needed.

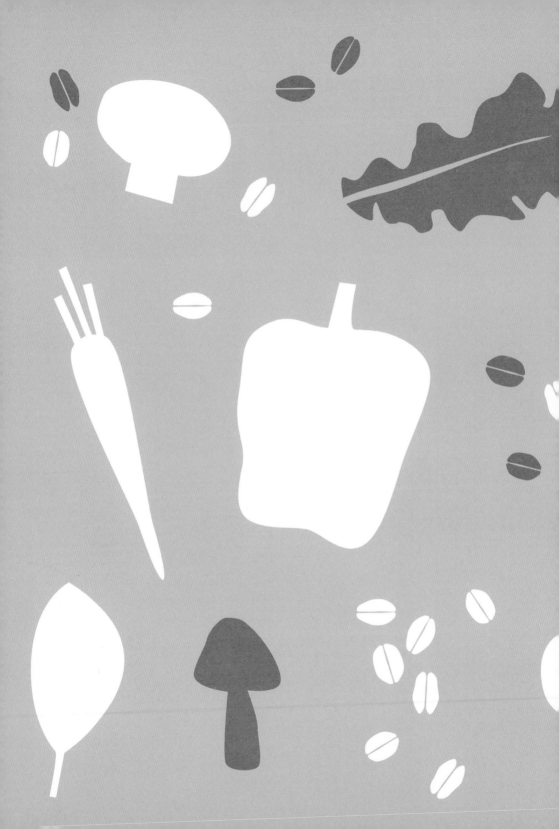

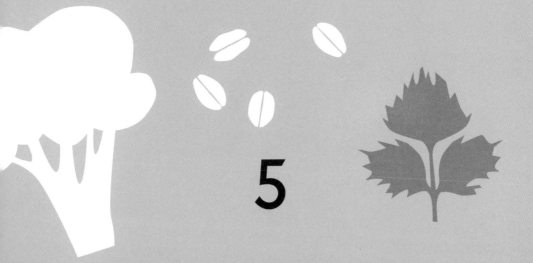

WHAT
DO I DO
WHEN... ?

5

What do I do when... ?

I want to try baby-led weaning, but I'm nervous of baby choking.
This is a very common concern for parents. You don't need to choose one method of feeding your baby; a gentle, combined approach to weaning works for many parents. Offering some soft finger foods, alongside some mashed foods or puree from a spoon can really work well. When it comes to offering finger foods make sure you start super-soft – try overcooking vegetables before offering them to baby and make sure that you can squidge them easily between your finger and thumb (see page 40).

My baby won't sleep through the night... will solids help?
The simple answer to this is no. Babies wake during the night for many reasons and, although there is a common misconception that weaning them early may help them to sleep better, this is not necessarily the case. If you feel your baby is ready for solid foods before around six month of age, have a chat with your health visitor and make sure baby is getting enough milk throughout the day. Don't forget to look out for the signs of readiness for weaning (see page 20), before you start offering solid foods to your baby.

My baby was born premature – should we wait to wean?
Sometimes premature babies may take a little longer to develop the skills needed for eating, and their weaning progress may take a little more time. However, most of the guidelines around weaning babies generally are still relevant. Ideally get support from your healthcare professional and look out for those signs of readiness (see page 20); these are still essential, but may simply come at different times. Check out the fantastic guidance on Bliss.org.uk for further information and support on weaning premature babies.

When it comes to offering my baby yoghurt… which type should I choose?
Plain, natural or Greek yoghurt are all good options for babies and toddlers. Choose full-fat options as babies need energy-dense foods. It's always best to opt for natural varieties when it comes to dairy, rather than flavoured yoghurts or yoghurts with added sugars; babies don't need the added sugar and, once they've been offered sweeter yoghurts, they may be less likely to accept the plain varieties. If you are worried about dairy allergies, see page 56.

Everyone tells me I should start weaning with baby rice?
This is a common question and the answer is really up to you. I recommend a veg-led approach to weaning, starting with a single taste of a different vegetable each day. You can start with baby rice if you prefer, but you absolutely don't have to. Baby rice can be used as a filler for some of the vegetable purees I recommend. Just be sure to choose a baby rice that is plain, with no added salt or sugar.

My baby doesn't seem to like vegetables… do I keep offering them?
It's not unusual for babies not to take to the taste of vegetables right away. Research shows that familiarisation is what leads to acceptance, which is why it's recommended to start vegetables early in the weaning process. If your baby hasn't taken to some of the vegetables you've offered in the first 10 days, that's OK. Continue to build on the variety of foods your baby has, but don't give up on vegetables. Keep gently offering them to baby in different forms and along with a variety of other foods. It can take up to 10 offerings before some foods are accepted – sometimes even longer (see page 34). Importantly, don't force or pressure your baby to eat foods they aren't accepting.

I'm unsure about giving certain foods (ground nuts/fish/lentils/meat/egg/spinach/spices) when my baby seems so young?

Most foods are fine to offer to baby in moderation and in variety from six months of age. I often get asked about certain foods such as ground seeds, ground nuts, lentils, herbs and spices for babies. ALL the foods you need to avoid initially are listed on page 56. Remember to offer foods gradually to baby, especially allergens or strong-tasting foods and spices.

My baby is rejecting the spoon. What do you suggest?

Often after initial acceptance of the spoon, some babies just go off it and will clamp their mouth shut. If this happens to your little one, know that it's common and it's also OK. It's often a phase and may simply be a sign of your baby showing that they want their own independence around eating. Try focusing on finger foods at mealtimes, but don't give up the spoon. Try loading a spoon for them and pop it next to them so they can begin to pick it up and feed themselves.

My baby is throwing food.

This is such a common complaint from parents as the weaning journey progresses. Babies inevitably like to play and experiment – it's all part of their learning and skill development. And that often involves throwing and dropping foods! Most of the time this is just a phase, as baby explores their environment and gravity, so try not to get too stressed about it and just know that this stage will pass. To ensure it isn't a prolonged phase, you can try the following:

* Don't draw too much attention to it – the more attention given, the more likely they will be to do it again.
* Invest in a floor mat or use an old tablecloth to protect the floor. You can then also pick food up and offer it again to baby.
* Pick up thrown or dropped food without much comment, maybe a little 'No, this isn't what we do with food', but no more than that ideally.
* Role model and show baby what we DO do with food.
* Have a side plate for 'unwanted' food and ask/show baby to use this instead of the floor.

My baby hasn't taken to weaning at all. We are a month in and no food has gone in?

All babies progress through weaning at very different paces. The information in this book is a guide and will vary hugely from child to child. Try not to compare your baby to others. If your baby isn't accepting solids well, have a chat with your health visitor and see if there may be an underlying reason for this. You could also consider the following:

* Baby's current milk intakes – if large amounts are being consumed (especially around mealtimes) this may affect their appetite.
* The eating environment – is baby calm, awake and relatively happy when you start mealtimes? If not, can you change up the environment so that baby is in more of a calm mood before you begin (see page 48)?
* Are you eating with your baby? This can make a huge difference to how a baby progresses through weaning, as they learn by watching you.
* Are mealtimes structured? Without a routine some babies can be reluctant to take foods at mealtimes as they don't know what to expect.
* Avoid pressuring baby to eat – this will often have the opposite effect. Try to make mealtimes enjoyable, pressure-free environments. Never force a baby to eat.

Offering my baby snacks… How many snacks does my baby need?

Babies don't really need any snacks until they are around one year old, and even then, their need for snacks may be determined by the rest of their diet. Before 12 months, try to make sure your baby is having three balanced meals a day and offer milk feeds in between. Allowing baby to graze or snack on other food throughout the day may affect their appetite for mealtimes. Once baby gets to 12 months of age, snacks may form a beneficial part of their food routine. Snacks can be a way to add extra nutrients and calories into baby's diet, so try to choose nutrient-rich snacks and think about them as 'mini-meals' rather than simply offering a yoghurt or a biscuit. Check out 'Balancing baby's meals' on page 114 and try the 'Finger foods, light bites and puds' ideas on pages 185–193.

When it comes to fruit and veg… do I need to buy organic?

If you want to buy organic, please do, but don't feel under pressure. Research suggests that organic food isn't necessarily any more nutrient-rich than standard produce, but lower levels of pesticides and artificial fertilisers are used when growing or processing organic produce. It's ultimately an individual choice for parents. With any vegetables and fruits, wash them well and use as fresh as possible for maximum nutritional benefits.

INDEX

FURTHER READING

NHS: Introducing solid foods to baby information from the UK's National Health Service: www.nhs.uk/conditions/pregnancy-and-baby/solid-foods-weaning

BSACI: Infant feeding and allergy prevention factsheet for parents: www.bsaci.org/wp-content/uploads/2020/02/pdf_Infant-feeding-and-allergy-prevention-PARENTS-FINAL-booklet.pdf

Ellyn Satter: *Child of Mine: Feeding with Love and Good Sense* www.ellynsatterinstitute.org

Keep a Beat UK: For information on baby first aid www.keepabeat.com

Leap Study: One of two major trials looking at earlier introduction of allergens to a baby during weaning: www.leapstudy.co.uk

Eat Study: One of two major trials looking at earlier introduction of allergens to a baby during weaning: www.ncbi.nlm.nih.gov/pmc/articles/PMC4852987

WITH THANKS

I want to say a HUGE thank you to my friends and family who have supported me in so many ways with this book. I'd be here all day listing you all, but thank you for trying recipes, babysitting, reading segments and supporting me through this project.

I also want so say a BIG thank you to Joe Wicks, without whom I may not be in this position in my career. Joe has been so kind to me and a really inspirational mentor. Thank you Joe.

Thanks to my Instagram audience, without whom I wouldn't have as much knowledge as I have today. Your questions each day drive me to learn and grow as a nutritionist and for that, and the kind words and support, I'm very grateful.

My colleagues also need a big shout out – nutritionists, dietitians, health visitors, speech and language therapists and first aiders – who have helped ensure that this book is as evidence-based, practical and helpful for parents as can be. Thank you, especially to Claire Baseley, Penny Barnard, Charlie Blyth, Paula Hallam and Stacey Zimmels.

Thanks to all the team at Penguin, including the editors, publishers, photographers and stylists for all your help in putting this together. I'm so glad you believed in what I wanted to create and helped me to get it just right.

Lastly, a HUGE thank you to my son, Raffy, who really has made all this possible and been my little model/recipe tester/ guinea pig throughout – thank you for making weaning and feeding fun for us all and for being you – funny, mad and everything in between!

1

Vermilion, an imprint of Ebury Publishing,
20 Vauxhall Bridge Road,
London SW1V 2SA

Vermilion is part of the Penguin Random
House group of companies whose
addresses can be found at global.
penguinrandomhouse.com

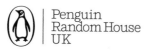
Penguin
Random House
UK

First published by Vermilion in 2021

www.penguin.co.uk

A CIP catalogue record for this book is
available from the British Library

Commissioning Editor: Sam Jackson
Project Editor: Emma Owen
Designer: Studio Polka
Photographer: Haarala Hamilton
Food Stylist: Frankie Unsworth

ISBN 9781785043246

Printed and bound in China by
C&C Offset Printing Co., Ltd

The authorised representative in the
EEA is Penguin Random House Ireland,
Morrison Chambers, 32 Nassau Street,
Dublin D02 YH68.

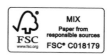

Penguin Random House is committed
to a sustainable future for our business,
our readers and our planet. This book is
made from Forest Stewardship Council®
certified paper.